Condition to

WIN

Dynamic Techniques for Performance Oriented Mental Conditioning

WES DOSS

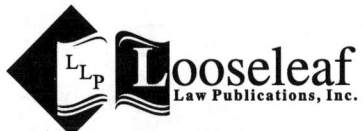

43-08 162nd Street
Flushing, NY 11358
www.LooseleafLaw.com
800-647-5547

This publication is not intended to replace nor be a substitute for any official procedural material issued by your agency of employment or other official source. Looseleaf Law Publications, Inc., the author and any associated advisors have made all possible efforts to ensure the accuracy and thoroughness of the information provided herein but accept no liability whatsoever for injury, legal action or other adverse results following the application or adoption of the information contained in this book.

10-digit: ISBN 1-932777-37-7
13-digit: ISBN 978-1-932777-37-6

Library of Congress Cataloging-In-Publication Data

Doss, Wes.
 Condition to win : dynamic techniques for performance oriented mental conditioning / Wes Doss.
    p. cm.
 Includes index.
 ISBN-13: 978-1-932777-37-6
 1. Physical fitness. 2. Physical fitness--Psychological aspects. 3. Mental discipline. I. Title.
 GV481.D67 2007
 613.7--dc22

                              2006036556

TABLE OF CONTENTS

DEDICATION

To those who have gone forth into harm's way and stared into the eyes of a dedicated opponent and walked away the victor and for those who gave all and never returned.

To my wife, Hye Chong, the driving force behind all I do, my love, my life and my best friend, I love you.

To my greatest heroes, living as examples of never giving up and working through any problems thrown at them, my two daughters, Angela and Victoria.

ABOUT THE AUTHOR

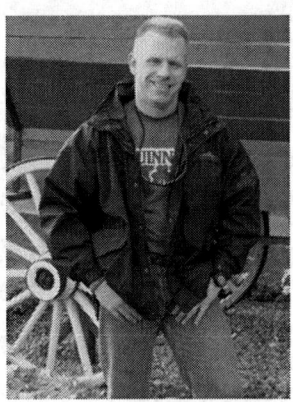

Wes Doss, near his home
in Northern Arizona

Wes Doss is an internationally recognized firearms, tactics, use of force and force application instructor with over 20 years of military and civilian criminal justice experience, as well as significant operational time with both military and law enforcement tactical operations and protective service organizations. Wes holds specialized instructor certifications from the U.S. Army, the U.S. Marine Corps, Arizona POST, the Smith & Wesson Academy, the Sigarms Academy, the NRA LEAD, and FEMA.

Wes has studied adult education and human performance extensively and has a broad background in the martial arts, with over 25 years of training, teaching, full contact and MMA/NHB fighting experience. Wes is the founder, President, and General Operating Manager of Khyber Interactive Associates, LLC and holds a Master's degree in Criminal Justice Administration and a Bachelor's degree in psychology. Wes is a member of a number of professional associations, including: The International Association of Law Enforcement Firearms Instructors (IALEFI), The American Society of Law Enforcement Training (ASLET), The National Rifle Association (NRA), The National Tactical Officers Association (NTOA), The Military Police Regimental Association (MPRA), and the International Association of Counter Terrorism and Security Professionals (IACTSP).

Wes is also a published author, with numerous articles in various publications, such as:

SWAT magazine
ASLET "The Trainer"
The NTOA "Tactical Edge"
Tactical Equipment Review
Tactical Gear
Police
Law Officer
American Cop

Wes is also the author of the book "Train to Win," a training psychology/philosophy book focused on law enforcement and military trainers and professionals.

ACKNOWLEDGMENTS

"You will never be a leader unless you first learn to follow and be led."

— Tiorio

A book like this one wouldn't be possible without the input and inspiration of others. I want to take just a brief opportunity to thank a few of those who inspired me to complete this second book.

Robert Taylor
The Taylor Group
(Prince George County
(MD) Police Ret.)

Steven "Chief" Bronson
Tactical Waterborne
Operations (USN Ret.)

Clyde Caceres
First Light USA

Sgt. James L. Gallagher
Boston (MA) Police Dept.

Al Baker
Baker Bat Shield
(NYPD ESU Ret.)

Sal Mascoli
Las Vegas (NV)
Metro Police Dept.

Ken Murray
Armiger Police Training
Institute

Michael de Bethencourt
Northeast Tactical
Schools

Nick Iltsopoulos
Spartacus Security

David S. Smith
"JD 'Buck' Savage"
(Arizona DPS Ret.)

Jim Cirrilo
(NYPD Stakeout
squad Ret.)

Dep. Jennifer
Fulford-Salvano
Orange Co. (FL)
Sheriff's Office

Ofc. Jarrod King
Alexandria (LA) Police
Department

Marc Scott
Controlled Tactical
Solutions

Special Thanks

For creative influence, design, and photo support I want to thank the following people.

Perry Taylor
Creative Concepts
Photography

Mark Burnell
SG5

Upendra Thapa

INTRODUCTION

"I know the price of success: dedication, hard work and an unremitting devotion to the things you want to see happen."

– Frank Lloyd Wright

Have you ever tried to build something detailed like a building or house? Consider a contractor getting ready to start a new project, like building or remodeling a house. First the contractor must make sure he has measurements and plans for the job. Next he would contact a building supply store and order the necessary supplies. Finally he would gather together all the necessary tools and manpower for the job and then start the job. Can you imagine trying to build the project with nothing but a screwdriver or hammer? In force application training we are making a similar mistake, if all the tools required for success are not on hand.

Year after year police officers, soldiers and other armed professionals spend considerable time on the range or on the mats working on the mechanical techniques of their trade. It is often the case, however, that the mind is not trained along with the body.

With the current tempo of today's world and its various high risk challenges, it could be beneficial to start utilizing mental skills in conjunction with the mechanical skills. *Condition to Win* is designed to be a resource for trainers, operators, and administrators. The information contained in it is both a practical and useful tool for individuals responsible for training personnel at all levels in law enforcement, military and security roles.

Due to the nature of this text and its intended audience, the order of the chapters has been carefully determined. The first half of the manual addresses **practical** and **foundational skills** and the remainder of the manual focuses on **performance skills**. These are more complex skills that build on the foundation created by the practical and foundational skills.

Mental skills are as real and as valuable as any other skill. Mental skills are equivalent to physical and mechanical skills in that they are all skill sets that must be learned and eventually contribute to the utmost in performance. However, most of the time trainers and operators view mental skills as something that an individual either has or doesn't have. Frequently dismissing their value and misunderstanding how to apply and cultivate them.

Mental skills and mental training are not the exclusive domain of elite warriors, like Navy SEALs, Army Special Forces, or Marine Force Recon. They also represent a critical training and skill component that is invaluable in the lives and careers of all who face violence by choice or as a condition of employment. Like any skill, mental skills must be cultivated and practiced. This action leads to a strong foundation that is an important component of both training and operational situations. Without mental training, operators often fail to spot opportunities that can lead to success or missed situational cues that could have prevented tragedy: physically prepared, but not mentally ready.

Mental training is not a simple process, even though we all have the ability to learn and manage situations internally. However, many individuals fail to develop their mental skills fully, due primarily to an unwillingness to train the mind and the body simultaneously. These are individuals who tend to be inconsistent...some good performances and many incidents of not-so-good performances. Individuals who make the effort to train the mind recognize that this type of conditioning takes time, effort and persistence, just like physical training.

Although most trainers and operators consider mental skills an important facet of well-rounded training, not all individuals and trainers have access to a mental skills specialist (sports or performance psychologist). However, trainers, who interact routinely with those in their charge, can serve as mental skills facilitators, helping to provide direction, guidance and support. *Condition to Win* was created, in part with my first book *Train to Win*, to aid trainers in conditioning their students and incorporating mental skills into their own training regimes.

The Realities of Performance Psychology

Performance Psychology can:

- Increase an operator's ability to remain in control under high levels of pressure.
- Increase an operator's performance consistency.
- Help operators perform at their best ability in training and under operational conditions.

Performance Psychology cannot:

- Replace physical training.
- Replace technical or mechanical skills training.
- Increase an operator's physical potential.

Bringing Performance Psychology to your Students

In this text, every chapter stands on its own and you are not required to instruct every skill. However, I suggest that as opportunities present themselves, you conduct mental training sessions and you introduce different skills to your students.

When you opt to begin using mental skills training in your own training regimen, you will need to discuss with them the key points that have been highlighted earlier in this section:

1. Importance of addressing mental skills
2. The need to consistently cultivate and practice mental skills
3. Mental skills are not easy
4. What performance psychology can and cannot do

In conjunction with introducing the new concept of mental skills, steps should also be taken to integrate it with the physical and mechanical skills currently being taught. Following the initial training, operators should be reminded several times about using their new mental skills in both training and real world events.

Good Luck!

Chapter One

WHY MENTAL TRAINING?

"Mental toughness is essential to success."
— Vince Lombardi

T he protectors: law enforcement, military, or security are for all intents and purposes members of a warrior class. Though this is not a politically correct view, it is both an accurate and realistic one. Having followed the calling to safeguard the lives and well-being of others, these rare individuals are certainly much more a warrior class than the professional athletes who are often considered in this elite status. The more specialized these warriors become, the more elite they are considered.

An elite warrior is a rare combination of drive, preparation, and the right frame of mind. In the real world of today and the unknown of tomorrow, we are inundated with a plethora of training principles and programs, some good, some bad and have unrestricted access to the best facilities and equipment available. Often, the real difference between the good and the elite or the survivors and the winners are the developed mental qualities of the warrior. The focus of this tome is on conditioning, harnessing anxiety and cultivating internal motivation. All aimed at winning, not merely surviving...**Train to Win!**

The Mind or Minds

Although we have one brain, we truly have two distinctly different minds: the conscious and the subconscious. The conscious mind relies on logic, deduction and reasoning to reach conclusions and to make decisions. The choices that we face, the decisions as to what we will or will not do are made through the conscious mind, not the subconscious mind. However, when we learn how to pass the conscious mind and allow the subconscious to act, we allow our conscious mind to be guided and influenced by the abilities of the subconscious mind. The subconscious mind

1

does not think or act on its own volition or initiative. The primary purpose of the subconscious mind is to achieve the goals that have been set by the conscious mind.

Without establishing goals to reach or facing problems to solve, we fail to load the subconscious mind for performance. But if we do give it goals and objectives, determined through experience, the subconscious mind will do what it is designed to do.

The various researches conducted in the fields of anatomy, physiology, and applied psychology; those involved in the field of human performance have come to understand that the subconscious mind functions like a computer, with its various functions dictated by the conscious mind, only much more complicated and intricate than any man-made piece of computer equipment. Even if a computer could be built as sophisticated, as complex and as detailed as the subconscious mind, it would still require a conscious human mind to operate it. A man-made computer does not have a built-in conscious mind to direct its actions, nor does it pose original problems to itself. It has no imagination, no creativity, and cannot set its own goals. Further, it has no emotions to help it face moral decisions or hold it back. The man-made computer only operates on the data supplied to it from an outside, human source.

The subconscious mind operates less rapidly and less accurately, in some respects, compared to a man-made computer, primarily because it is human and not a machine and therefore subject to all the thoughts and emotions of the conscious mind. As a simple example of how the conscious mind directs the subconscious, let's look at the simple action of feeding ourselves. We accomplish this simple goal because of a set habitual pattern that we have programmed into our subconscious through repetitive action. Although early on, as small children, we had a difficult time hitting our mouths with our food, by our adulthood we no longer rely on our conscious mind to tell the subconscious to move the fork from the plate to the mouth. It also does not have to tell the body which muscles to use to accomplish this task. The subconscious mind has been programmed through prior experience and conditioning to perform the movements without any action from the conscious mind. The purpose of this simple example is to show that once a correct or successful response has been established in the subconscious mind, it allows it to attain the specific goals given it with the conscious mind; the procedure is stored and maintained for future use.

The subconscious mind repeats this successful response, as well as failures in some cases, on future trials, no matter what they are. It has learned to respond because that is what the conscious mind has directed it to do. The subconscious remembers its successes, usually discarding failures, so long as it recognizes them as failures, and repeats those actions as a matter of habit without any further thought or direction from the conscious mind. In fact, certain habit patterns become so deeply ingrained in the subconscious mind that the goals given to it by the conscious mind can be easily accomplished, in the dark or with the eyes closed. However, when a skill or response is not supported with a sense of confidence, or the individual doubts his or her abilities, especially under periods of high stress or demand, the conscious mind tries its best to "back seat drive" and take control from the subconscious mind. The competition in control is often characterized as "choking" and it can be a fatal competitive event. The key is developing the subconscious mind with the right information, the right skills, and the right responses and then maintaining the right level of confidence and belief in it, allowing those responses to be automatic and reflexive, keeping the conscious mind out of the way of the subconscious.

The conscious mind is that part of the brain often termed "the active brain" and it enables you to know, think and act effectively. The conscious mind uses logic, deduction and reasoning to reach conclusions and make decisions. Choices and decisions as to what you will or will not do are made in the conscious mind. The conscious mind takes cognizance of the objective world around us. Its method of observing the environment is through the use of the body's five physical senses: sight, smell, sound, touch and taste. We gain knowledge through these senses. The conscious mind learns through observation, experience and education. In contrast, the subconscious mind is completely impersonal and does not have the capacity of making moral judgments or determining the difference between right and wrong, good or evil. The subconscious mind is designed to work automatically and impersonally to achieve goals, regardless of whether those goals are good or evil, right or wrong, moral or immoral. While the conscious mind relies on our physical senses, the subconscious mind seems to respond off the less popular sixth sense or intuition.

To give this perspective, let me relate a simple and humorous personal story to illustrate this point. Several years ago, the U.S. Army sent me to Camp Williams just outside of Salt Lake City, Utah, for training. At the end of our exhaustive training evolution, the class was allowed the opportunity to leave post and spend some time in Salt Lake City blowing off steam. Well, like any bunch of little kids in big bodies, this meant we were going to spend time drinking and telling war stories. Several hours later and into the wee hours of the Utah morning, my compatriots and I began slowly making our way back to post for our morning formation. We had a rental car and I sat in the back seat with two other soldiers, I sat on the driver's side. Now it is important to note that I am the father of two very beautiful girls who are in their teens. During their younger ages we would take family trips in the car to visit relatives or go on vacation and as any father of small children knows, children in moving vehicles often expel stomach contents for no real reason and when they do they initiate that action with some very obvious visual and audible cues, that to a non-parent may go unnoticed. On the ride back to post the passenger in the middle of the tight-cramped back seat uttered a low guttural gurgle that caused my subconscious to fly into action. I quickly pivoted in my seat, forcing the middle passenger up against the guy on the passenger side. Almost immediately the middle passenger vomited with the force and glory of the final days of Pompeii. Because of my actions, I was spared the mess and embarrassment of getting heaved on by a fellow soldier. The guy on the passenger side did not fare so well. The point here is that my entire action was from the subconscious, because some part of me recognized the sound and associated it with the nasty semi-digested contents of the stomach. I acted and ultimately won.

Winning as a Warrior

Since the subconscious mind can't tell right from wrong, it is always important for us to frame ourselves with the material to allow us to act in the most appropriate way possible. This means developing a winning attitude, looking at the actions required of us in high demand, high risk situations, the way elite athletes look at high demand sporting events. By embracing this approach, we take significant steps toward the skills needed to keep our head in the game, maintain emotional control to maximize effectiveness and mitigate the negative influences of fear and anxiety on our performance. To get us started in the right direction, I want each of you to consider your role as the protector, as a member of a true warrior class. Stop considering your occupation as just a job and look more at the higher calling that it truly is. If you're a trainer, your calling is even higher. It is your exclusive honor to share your knowledge and skills and shape the lives and actions of other warriors.

Who and What Is a Warrior?

You will no doubt notice that I use the term "warrior" throughout this book to describe the men and women that protect us, defend us and sacrifice so much for our personal freedoms and our way of life. It is important for our modern warriors to understand their role in society and accept it, come to terms with it and understand all the details the occupation has. This has become increasingly more difficult, as the nature of our occupations has grown more administrative and litigious (a nice way of saying kinder and gentler—touchy-feely).

The warrior, throughout history, was a spiritual soul, one who was only incidentally concerned with warfare; the Samurai of medieval Japan administered a peaceful government and maintained a high level of personal discipline and integrity and the American Indian warriors exercised ritualistic combat that represented exercises in bravery rather than death. In fact, many "wars" between tribal factions did not result in fatalities. The focus of these warriors was to live and maintain harmony. A central theme of service existed as warriors of the day were the defenders of societal values, and maintained their own personal values of courage, loyalty, selflessness, service and guardianship (Heckler, 2000).

Traditional warriors of history often found themselves much more concerned with conflict than they preferred, because technology of the day was not advanced enough to farm where farms did not exist or establish other methods of world-wide transportation. It was easier to simply invade a land and take what *they* had as your own. Because of this, much of the world's early societies were constantly in a state of war. While members of early societies were probably no more intrinsically violent than members of today's modern societies, they accepted, often celebrating, the use of force as a final conciliator of human and societal affairs. Until the time when laws became paramount in the minds of men, might literally meant right and in inter-personal or inter-societal terms, this equated to endless war.

In early societies, warfare was not only considered a man's business, but it was the most significant factor in life throughout the world. Warfare was an occupation of a great many adult males, for which they trained from early childhood. This training typically began with initiation ceremonies marking the exit from childhood and entrance into adulthood, separating the warrior from women and children.

There was a strong sense of individualism among early traditional warriors, the honor achieved in conflict being primarily individual honor, won through personal valor in lieu of group success. Trophies, in the form of scalps or skulls, were important. Fighting as individuals, even as part of an army, in very close quarters, the early warrior knew exactly who had triumphed and by what means. Victory was generally a personal matter and the trophies collected were a testimony of that individual success.

The motives of conflict were pragmatic. In North American cultures, for example, social stratification was primarily military, and success on the battlefield was how a man attained social status. Success in war was also how a man gained advancement; war honors were public tokens of courage and ability and, as such, were regarded as credentials for societal positions. Even in the early days of our own country, war heroes and leaders were considered to be outstanding choices for the political theater.

The ancient Greeks changed the philosophical principle and introduced a sense of morality or higher purpose to conflict. It was they who first believed that combat ennobles the human spirit, and that man's highest values—courage, endurance, skill, and sacrifice—could be experienced only in conflict. The Greek notion of dying fearlessly, sword in hand, facing the enemy, has been integral to the warrior's self-image for most of recorded Western history. Homer, Hector and Achilles all articulated the concept of "heroic warfare" in their various works of literature.

The Knight

From earliest times, Europe was an amalgamation of warrior societies, the "armies" met and defeated by the Roman legions consisted of all the able men of a tribe or people who fought as infantry: On foot, with spear, sword, and shield. In the years following the decline of the Roman Empire (about 400 AD), there was a great technological evolution. By the eighth and ninth centuries, the only fighting man of any real consequence was the mounted warrior, the knight.

During the Norman Conquest in 1066, knights were nothing more than warriors trained to fight from horseback. They were men held on retainer or in service to someone of nobility. The concept of the knight morphed over time as the tools and goals of war evolved. From being the obligation of every able adult male, warrior status narrowed to where it only pertained to an elite class of men. Eventually, producing an aristocratic class that enjoyed an elevated status in society and like other warriors, medieval knights fought individually and put their personal honor, fame and fortune above all else.

The Samurai

In Japan, the samurai began and ended the same way as the knights. The concept of the samurai was first applied to personal attendants who were nothing more than domestic servants. It later came to refer to the class of warriors who attended the provincial landowners in the tenth and eleventh centuries. Regardless of how populous the battlefield, the early samurai, much like the knights, fought individually against single opponents, primarily an opponent of similar rank, skill and merit.

The samurai extended total loyalty to his immediate overlord while at the same time looking to his own advantage. He fought alone and engaged in personal heroics in order to impress his lord. The relationship between the lord and the samurai echoed the bond of the knight and his lord, but more extreme since it ranked higher than the bonds of family. Like the knight, the samurai's powerful confidence was fed by a strong belief system; in the samurai's case, this was Zen Buddhism and the warrior code of Bushido. Under these influences, which place a premium on discipline and self-control, samurai theorists insisted that the true warrior must be constantly prepared to make the ultimate sacrifice for his lord, without a moment's reflection or conscious consideration.

**WARRIOR: A man engaged or experienced in war;
a soldier; a champion.**

Webster's Dictionary

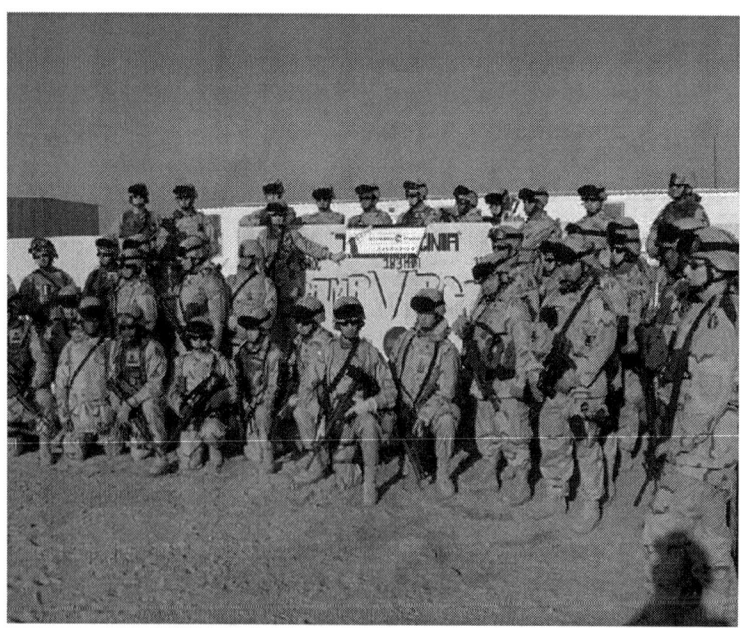

While the legendary Samurai and Knights of the middle ages are gone, one does not have to look too far to find elite warriors today.

Do knights and samurai exist today? No. Not in the form that the words conjure in the minds of the listener or reader. Do Warriors exist in today's world? Absolutely! Being a Warrior, being of a mindset that would enable one to fight or function in harsh or critical situations, is achievable even in our modern occupations and societies. It is a matter of focus, dedication, wisdom and honor. And... because of these requirements, it is not for everyone. It is important to understand that while mechanical and mental skills can be developed in anyone, not everyone is built for conflict. Warriors may come from any walk of life, sharing in the internal soul which makes them excel at what they choose to do. They will rise above those around them, and will be better prepared to handle challenge and adversity.

Does being a soldier, Marine, sailor or law enforcement officer make one a Warrior? Absolutely not, not alone, anyway. Being a warrior is far from just a simple occupation, any more than it's about being a 6'4" and 240- pound bundle of anger—it's about making conscious choices about how you think. The development of the warrior is a combination of real confidence, detailed concentration, and firm tenacity. However, those qualities are next to worthless, without the physical and mechanical skills to complete a task—but so, too, are the physical skills without mindset.

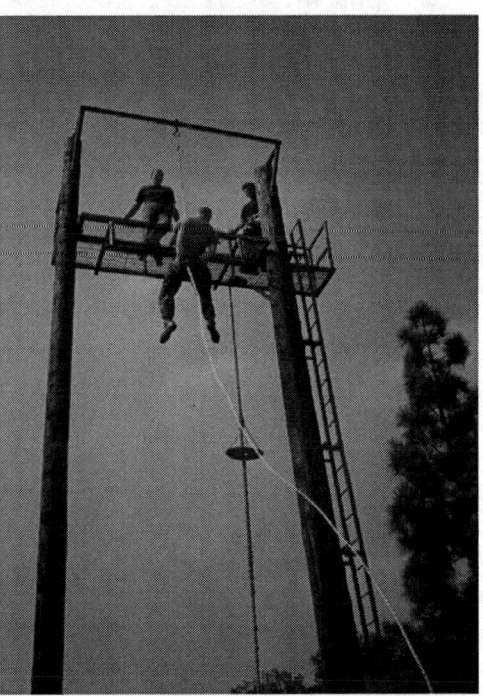

Cultivating skills of the warrior is no easy task, it requires skill, patience, and an understanding of the individual psychological dynamics that make up the warrior.

Mental skills are cultivated not by throwing people who can't swim into water, but by training and conditioning them to deal with extreme situations, by conditioning them to focus effectively, by teaching them the importance of confidence, and how to build and maintain personal confidence.

Why So Much Emphasis on Mental Training?

The human mind and its relationship to the body is undeniably strong. For literally every thought in your mind your body has some sort of physically response. It makes no difference if it's real or pure fantasy. Remember a bad dream? Ever wake up with your heart racing, sweating, angry or scared? Ever dream of eating something and wake up with the taste in your mouth? In the mind something was happening and the body, unable to discern fact from fiction, was reacting to the "event." Another example: you're walking through the dark woods at night and you hear something that gives you cause to feel afraid. Your mind interprets the noise as something to fear, perhaps an attacker or a wild animal. Once the emotion of fear sets in, the obligatory release of chemicals occurs to activate the SNS. These are just simple examples of how powerful the bond is between the mind and the body. With this understanding, it's not hard to see how critical it is to address both physical and mental training when we train for performance.

In the real world field of conflict, so many things are left to chance. Conflict is a predictably unpredictable medium. Why become part of that uncertainty? We all possess the power and ability to control this realm and to control ourselves. Warriors spend so much time physically and mechanically training in hopes of getting an edge on all potential opponents. However, most organizations and individuals forget about the most powerful performance enhancement tool. In fact, this powerful device is already in their possession. I am, of course, speaking about the mind. While it's commonly mentioned that skills are 90% mental and only 10% physical, it is far from common practice. The excuses given for not addressing mental training vary: lack of time, lack of resources, and even lack of belief. Whatever the reason, the fact remains, we are not utilizing our most powerful resource to its fullest capacity. Most people fatigue mentally long before they tire physically, due to the fact that the mind is not in as good a shape as the physical skills. In 1996, I and a bunch of like- minded fools, launched into a training odyssey in hopes of winning the inaugural masochistic celebration known as the eco-challenge. If you're not familiar with the eco-challenge, it is one of a large number of adventure or expedition-style races where teams race together from start to finish, non-stop for hundreds of miles over daunting terrain in hopes of winning a cash prize that isn't even close to the amount of time and energy put into preparing and competing in this type of event. I love it! During our training, weekend-long training sessions, we would typically run mini-races, often moving from event to event with no sleep; while our bodies had energy our minds fatigued. This fatigue often manifested itself as doubt, nervousness, fear and full-on hallucinations.

The odds of success in conflict are always tight; often the margin for domination is slim. Administrators, trainers and warriors are starting to understand that as society gets more violent and more skilled they need an edge, a new resource, a trained mind. However, many trainers are blind to the value of mental skills training for their warriors. When two opponents are physically and mechanically matched, it is the warrior who is mentally prepared and confident that will walk away victorious. However, it's important to never forget that no form of mental training will compensate for ineffective techniques or skills. In addition to mental preparation, warriors must be strong, technically and mentally. Unfortunately, many times, one aspect of training is magnified at the expense of the other. Attention must be given to all aspects of training; this is the ideal approach. You are a warrior or the trainer of warriors, perhaps both. You have skills and talent. It's your job to cultivate that proficiency by combining physical, mechanical and mental training. You want your warriors to be prepared mentally and physically, to be the absolute best, increasing the odds of success.

Testaments to Mental Training

The following testimonials reflect the experiences of our peers; warriors who have dealt with the demands of a high stress, high performance situation and have chosen to share them for the sole purpose of this book and for helping others. These are candid, first-person accounts and are largely unedited. They express both the situation and solutions addressed by mental performance training. They are from the heart and from real warriors who have been there. Warriors whom I am proud to call personal friends.

The War on Wise Street
Officer Jarrod King
Alexandria, LA Police Dept.

On February 20, 2003, the brave men of the Alexandria Louisiana Police Department's SRT met with a set of circumstances that would ultimately cost the lives of two of their members and change the lives of the surviving members forever. Because of the focused actions of key members of the SRT, the tables were turned on a violent suspect, resolving the situation and saving lives.

The incident on Wise street was predicated a few days earlier with a "routine" armed robbery in a predominantly low-income section of Alexandria and responding officers Michael Fuller and his shift commander. The two officers searched the area, but were ultimately unsuccessful in locating the suspect. The shift commander left the area, but Officer Fuller remained. Sitting in his patrol car working on paperwork, Officer Fuller begins to take rounds from an unknown location in the neighborhood. 18 to 20 rounds were fired at Officer Fuller's vehicle, shattering windows and shredding metal. Fuller was able to take immediate evasive action and drive away, escaping serious injury. This incident started a two-day long campaign by the Alexandria Police Department to locate the suspect before further incidents.

The Alexandria PD's SRT was activated to provide protection to investigators in the field, working the ambush scene and as a show of force in the financially-recessed area that included Wise street. Detectives went door to door with SRT team members in an intense effort to bring closure to the incident. The investigation began to point to a specific suspect, Anthony Molette. Molette, a 25-year-old man with an arrest record that included a considerable number of violent crimes, including:

attempted murder, assault and battery. As the investigation began to narrow on Molette, the word was from the sources on the street that Molette was aware of the situation and the intense manhunt that was closing on him. Vowing he would not go back to prison, his intention was to "Hold court on Wise Street."

The Alexandria Police Department decided to execute a high risk warrant on Molette at his residence on February 19, but their search for Molette met with negative results and failed to turn up any evidence linking Molette to the shooting. The investigation continued and ultimately led the Police to 2316 Wise Street. In an overabundance of intelligence obtained from a number of sources, the Police department was able to surmise that Molette was in one of the many structures on the property and that he was heavily armed, but some confusion was created over stories that Molette may have others with him, including children. The only thing that was for sure was that Molette knew the SRT was on its way to find him and he was ready for them. During the execution of the warrant service for Molette, arriving officers and members of the SRT found themselves trapped in a virtual ambush.

During the lengthy firefight that ensued while trying to take Molette into custody, two of the SRT members were fatally wounded. Molette was killed in the return of fire by the other members of the SRT. At the time of writing this book, the specific details and actions of both Molette and the SRT personnel were still part of an ongoing dispute, however it is important to note that even with two officers down, key individuals on the SRT acted with extreme selfless actions, risking their own lives to keep the team up and running. bringing the situation to conclusion.

Officer Jarrod King, a principal member of the Alexandria Police Department's SRT shared this with me concerning the incident on Wise Street and the value he placed on mental training.

Mental mindset training is probably the most neglected part of our training regimen. I did not realize how important that was as an operator, until my team's first officer-involved shooting. After that incident I took it upon myself to develop my mindset along with my other tactical skills. I began to program my mind and work with my teammates to do whatever it took to be a winner in a violent encounter. I prepared myself not to ever give up when the situation was at its worst because if I did I would be failing myself, my teammates, family, and the public that depends on law enforcement to be there when it counts.

That training paid off when our team was involved in a fierce gun battle with an individual during which two of our teammates were killed and three others wounded. I know today that if I or any of my teammates had told ourselves, "I can't go on, this is too bad," we would have suffered many more casualties and would not have been able to see the incident through to its conclusion. As police officers, soldiers or any other person in harm's way, we have to prepare ourselves to win. The cost is too much to pay for us to lose.

Officer Jarrod King
Alexandria LA Police Department

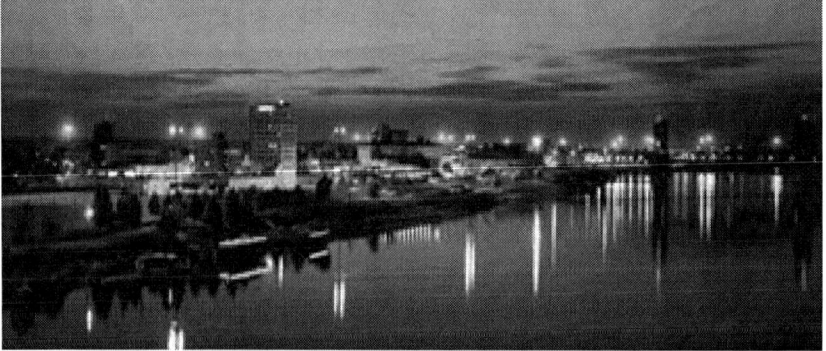

Alexandria, Louisiana, sits on the banks of the Red River in central Louisiana. A cultural crossroads in the South.

"I wasn't going to die there"
Deputy Jennifer Fulford-Salvano,
Orange County, FL Sheriff's Dept.

May 05, 2004 started with a 911 call for help in Pine Hills, Florida. Dextin Allen, a 9-year-old boy and his 2-year-old sister were trapped in their mother's mini-van in the garage of their home. Trapped there by the 3 gunmen who had invaded and occupied their home for the purpose of taking the more than 341 pounds of marijuana and $54,000 in cash that their father had hidden in the house.

Following the 911 call from 9-year-old Dextin, four Orange county deputies, Dwayne Martin, Kevin Curry, Jennifer Fulford, and Jason Gainor, were dispatched to the house. While en route, the officers were advised that the child had related to dispatch that there were "strange men" in his house and they were armed.

Deputies Martin and Curry were first on scene and initiated contact with a female at the home while Deputies Fulford and Gainor arrived. The woman turned to Deputy Fulford directly, presumably because she was the only female officer on scene. The woman told Deputy Fulford that her three children—9-year-old Dextin and his two-year-old twin sisters—were in the mini-van inside the garage of the home.

As the woman was told to wait at the street, the Deputies requested backup and K9 to respond. Deputies Gainor and Curry went to the opposite side of the residence. Deputy Fulford advised the other officers that she was going to check on the children in the minivan.

When Deputy Fulford entered the garage and walked up to the driver's side of the mini-van, she saw two small children buckled into car seats in the back and the doors of the van were locked. She suddenly heard male voices coming from the opposite side of the mini-van and then 3 to 4 gun shots from the same direction. Dropping to the ground, Deputy Fulford used her portable radio to notify others of "Shots Fired!" Not knowing the location of her fellow Deputies, she found herself trapped in the garage between the mini-van and an SUV—a space of less than

3 feet wide. A fraction of a second later a male came around the back of the mini-van and began firing at her.

Deputy Fulford immediately began returning fire with her .45 ACP caliber Glock 21 and the male suspect fell to the floor, but continued firing. Several rounds were exchanged and a second male appeared and began firing at her. Deputy Fulford maintained her ground, alternating rounds between her two targets. A short time after the male suspects began firing at her, Deputy Fulford realized that her legs had been hit several times and that she was losing blood. Deputy Fulford continued to shoot back and in her final exchange of fire with the male suspect at the rear of the mini-van, she delivered a fatal hit with a solid center mass hit, but not before he was able to hit her right arm, which was her dominant side, severely damaging it. Losing use of her dominant hand and arm, she switched to her left hand, a skill that had only recently been taught to her, and carried on the fight and exchanged shots with a second male suspect, ultimately shooting him and ending the situation.

During the gun fight, Deputy Fulford was struck 10 times—three rounds hit equipment, while seven rounds caused wounds on various parts of her body. According to the accounts of the officers and the dispatch log, the entire melee lasted 47 seconds. Subsequent investigation revealed that the suspects that had attacked Deputy Fulford had been trying to steal 341 pounds of marijuana and $54,000 in cash from the residents of the home. They had accosted the children and their mother as she was trying to take her kids to school and forced her back into the house, prompting the call by her son to police. When the gunmen realized that law enforcement had arrived, they told the women to go outside and tell the officers everything was OK and the call had been a mistake. When she didn't return, they planned to ambush the responding deputies with Glock 9mm and .40 caliber handguns.

While the quick response of all the deputies in this incident are noteworthy, the manner in which Dep. Fulford performed was awesome and stands as a tremendous example of the value of mindset development and mental conditioning. Deputy Fulford placed herself in harm's way, utilized her training and allowed developed skills in her subconscious to take control.

Dep. Fulford's actions earned her considerable notoriety, including Parade magazine's Police Officer of the Year and the International Association of Chiefs of Police Officer of the Year.

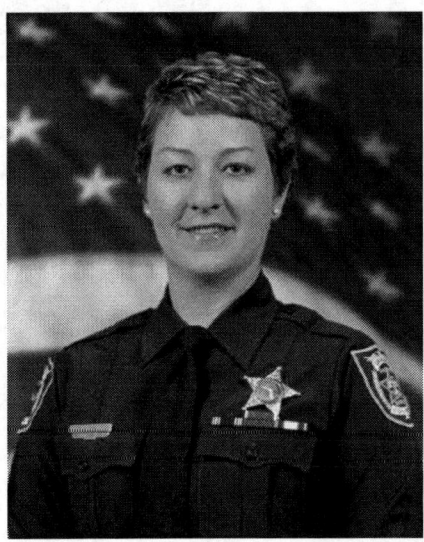

Dep. Jennifer Fulford-Salvano, of the Orange County (FL) Sheriff's Department; model police officer, true warrior, and my friend.

Mindset is one of the most important tools in keeping an officer alive during a deadly force encounter. Never convince yourself that you will die just because you get shot or injured. People have willed themselves to die after receiving injuries that should not have been fatal because that is what they believe is supposed to happen. Constantly running through scenarios relating to the calls that you encounter is essential. Get people together and perform mock simulations or at least run through the possible outcomes in your mind. I am sure that we have all heard, "Your body will not go where your mind has never been." If you have never thought about how you should react to various situations, you will be surprised when unexpected things happen. It has been proven that reaction is slower than action and having to think about how you should react to any given situation will significantly slow your response and could cost you your life.

No matter what happens, you MUST believe that you will not only live, but you will WIN. You must convince yourself that you can live through being shot, or stabbed, or run over, or whatever. You must believe that good (you) will triumph over evil (them) and that you will be the one going home to your family at the end of the day.

During an interview by the media, I was once asked if at any point I thought that I was not going to make it. I told them that was never an option. I would not have made it if I had let any doubts enter my mind. I believe that you must train hard and trust that it will kick in and get you through. Never doubt your ability to do your job or stay alive.

> Deputy Jennifer Fulford-Salvano,
> Orange County, FL Sheriff's Dept.

From a Dynamic Trainers View Point
Marc Scott, Controlled Tactical Solutions
Los Angeles, California

Marc Scott is a principal member of Controlled Tactical Solutions. Formed in 2002, Controlled Tactical Solutions, or CON-TACT Solutions, is a dynamic training organization dedicated to officer safety, effective technique, and training the legally justified in the use of force. CON-TACT Solutions has provided training and guidance for multiple local and federal law enforcement agencies.

Marc has an extensive history in training and conflict management. His martial arts training began somewhat differently than most. Although he had studied Judo and Tae Kwon Do as a child, it was as a teen that he was first exposed to the concept of functional martial skill. As a member of the Chinatown Pugilist Society in Ottawa, Canada, he was lucky enough to be exposed to a variety of instructors and teaching ideas in a non-traditional manner. Here he learned the elementary skills that he cultivated over years of training. Such things as grappling, boxing and stick and knife training were all par for the course in this early training. By the early nineties, Marc began to concentrate more on the idea of becoming an evolved fighter and finding out what worked and what didn't in a real context.

In 1993, Marc moved to the Czech Republic where he studied yet more martial arts, this time Di Pen Shi, a modern system of martial arts. By 1994, Marc had made the decision that to truly continue to grow as a martial artist and fighter he had to move outside of the circle with which he had been training. It was at this time that he made the first of many trips to Thailand to train and fight in Muay Thai kickboxing, renowned as one of the fiercest fighting styles in the world. He lived in Chiang Mai, Thailand where he trained twice a day, six days a week, learning the Muay Thai style until eventually he was given the right to teach and carry on the gym name outside of Thailand. This trip would prove a catalyst and Marc would continue to travel the world, training and competing, always absorbing as much of the local styles and systems of self-defense as possible. Life for Marc in the mid-nineties was a combination of time spent abroad and time in Canada, where he continued to train, this time with Igor Yakimov, Russian Sambo Champion and trainer to the Russian Military. Marc became a close, personal student and learned the devastating art of Russian Sambo. Marc continued his training with Igor and was certified as a full instructor in 2001. At present, Marc is the only fully certified instructor under Igor Yakimov.

As the century drew to a close, Marc was training and living in Thailand, Japan and Canada. It was in Japan that he was exposed to Shoot fighting, submission grappling, and Judo. For two years Marc lived and trained in Japan, competing in Shoot fighting and grappling competitions. From Japan Marc moved to the United States, where he began his training in Brazilian Jiu-Jitsu in earnest, as well as training for Mixed Martial Arts (MMA) competition. It was also there that he began to train with firearms and study modern pistol craft. During this time he worked as a doorman on the famed sunset strip in Los Angeles, getting plenty of opportunity to test his training in the real world.

Marc continued to develop his training methods and went outside the realm of civilian training. With time spent finding the needs of law enforcement and military, Marc went on to develop specific training methods for these groups. He developed systems that were implemented on the state and federal level, as well as being recognized by the United States Marine Corps as a Subject Matter Expert in edged weapon combat. It was in 2003 that Marc met and trained for the first time with Raymond Floro, a master of knife fighting who took the time to train Marc in his unique system of combat. Marc was certified by Raymond in 2004 and continues to explore and implement Floro Fighting Systems (FFS) into his training. In addition to his martial arts certifications, he is certified by the California Commission on Peace Officer Standards and Training, the Federal Emergency Management Agency, and the Red Cross.

All combat happens on two very different yet inter-twined levels, physical and mental. With either of these two aspects missing, your chance of success diminishes. As a trainer, I am cognizant of the fact that quite often we spend far more time on the physical than the mental. We are quick to dismiss mental training as not being as important or relevant to the work of the armed professional as physical skills development. There is a feeling that the mental toughness of the trainee is enough to carry him or her through any situation.

It was through Wes Doss that I first became exposed to the idea of how important mental training really is and how it related to the development of functional skills under real world conditions. All trainers face the dilemma creating as "real" a training environment as possible, and how to create as much useful stress as possible during it. Too much stress and you run the risk of mentally destroying the confidence of the trainee. Not enough stress and you allow the trainee to have an unrealistic expectation of combat which ulti-mately may crumble in the live theatre. In "Train to Win," Wes clearly outlined the importance of stress in training and how important it is in the development of functional skills. As a civilian Subject Matter Expert for the United States Marine Corps division schools, I have applied these methods across a wide variety of situations with hundreds of people with different levels of natural ability, and have found that the lessons Wes taught have led to an increase in learning, skill retention, and ability.

Marc Scott
Controlled Tactical Solutions
Los Angeles, California

Conditioning for Peak Performance

As I have previously discussed, this book is about conditioning for peak performance, the abilities that all warriors are trying to achieve and what training authorities are trying to help warriors, teams and organizations obtain. Since peak performance is the basis for the material in this book, let's look at some prevalent characteristics of the ultimate in performance. This way, you will have some understanding of these characteristics and concepts as you come across them repeatedly throughout the book.

Peak performance is often expressed as a "state of flow" or "being in the zone." Regardless of what it's called, it defines one single thing, that special phenomenon where you can do nothing wrong and everything goes right. A point in time when a warrior is so involved in what he or she is doing that nothing else seems to matter, a deep connection with the situation at hand. Unfortunately, these periods of optimum performance don't happen often enough. In fact, most times when it does happen, it is solely by chance. It just happened to be a day when everything just fell into place (Sugarman, 1991).

By implementing mental skills training and cultivating the skills developed, you can increase the frequency and consistency of zone or flow. Being in this state means doing more than anyone else ever thought possible, even exceeding your own expectations. This quest for zone or flow is why so many warriors are motivated in their own specific pursuits.

Driving Peak Performance for Warriors

Zone or flow (Ford & Marsh 1998) is a concept that relates to timing. It is most often described as "an optimal psychological state where complete absorption in a task at hand fosters a vast number of positive experiential events." Since several leading researchers maintain that zone and flow are necessary components for peak performance, especially under high stress or high demand events, a fair amount of research has been conducted in the area of zone and flow in an attempt to identify the various components of the process. Studies performed by these researchers suggest the presence of nine specific components in the activation of zone or flow:

1. Balance between the challenge and competence
2. Fusion between action and awareness
3. Clear objectives
4. Clear feedback
5. Focus
6. A sense of control
7. Loss of the sense of uncertainty
8. Temporal or chronological displacement
9. A sense of purpose

ak, 1990) that indicated that the effects of frustration
htecky, 1978), anxiety and worry (Adam & van Wieringen,
) enhances or aggravates tension, while deep relaxation
lander, Bergman & Archer, 1999), visualization (Harris &
nson, 1986) and self-talk (Harris & Robinson, 1986) reduces
on and mitigate aggravation. Bird (1987) described an
rimental case-study where an elite level 23-year-old rifle
sman demonstrated that the most successful performance
associated with ability to attain relatively low levels of
al activation. Between "taking-aim" and "firing," his level
xiety remained stable until an instant before firing, when it
nded sharply, rising again to normal level after firing.
r levels of anxiety during a series were associated with
r scores. Further, Janson (1995) reported a series of case-
es indicating that the most successful athletes within
ent disciplines (i.e., bowling, boxing, archery, discus, shot-
hammer, javelin, cycling, golf, marksmanship and weight-
) often produced lower anxiety levels, pre-, during- and
action, than less successful athletes, in each respective
this finding was confirmed even in the case of boxing
ably a technical activity). Janson (1995) noted, too, that
athletes show a markedly higher degree of synchronized
dance to arousal and anxiety to a much greater extent than
less skillful.

series of tests and studies were done by Norlander, Gård,
olm & Archer, in 2003, by interacting with elite athletes
a wide variety of disciplines and skill levels, including
ic level athletes. 33 specific categories were created and
c performances and experiences were related to each of the
ries. The 33 categories were derived from an analysis of
nd flow. A numeric scoring system of **Meaningful Units**,
s, was assigned to each category to determine its level of
ance or level of experience. Under each respective category
g is a short explanation of the category, and is followed by
oling of commentary from the test subjects.

W.D. Russell (2001) examined different qu
qualitative aspects of flow in 42 elite athletes
different team and individual sports and obtained
completely in agreement with the nine identifi
with regard to factors contributing to the zone ex
ever, Russell considered the situation incomplete
into consideration the dimensions that hinder
flow. In other words, those day to day occupatio
we allow to break our concentration and focus.

Jackson (1995) has suggested that factors di
rupting zone in athletes and warriors be conside
uncontrollable, at least the external ones. One
basic factor is "physical and mental readiness"
which is necessary for the coordination of all p
decisions and subsequent movements, thus als
flow and zone. This factor is also a condition
awareness to create a context thereby in line
factor. "Physical and mental readiness" may b
mind and body coordination to achieve timing
Benvenuti, Stanhope, Thomas, Panzer and Hal
Stein, 1999; Strauss & Klich, 1999). Studies
point to the obligation of considering the gender
gender differences may underlie intensity and
ment (Buchman, Leurgans, Gottlieb, Chen, Alr
2000).

Technical skill affects both timing and
Aggelousis, et al (2001) performed a study invc
aged 19–26 years, who were required to deve
throwing a ball. Analysis of four muscles in
showed that conditions allowing more trai
performance accompanied by reduced tensic
muscle and in the most important antagon
results confirmed those of an earlier study
done with children aged 7-11 where performa
through exercise was associated with reduc
muscles analyzed.

The power of psychological variables on
tension has been subjected to investigation

Sve
(Ry
198
(No
Rob
tens
expe
mar
was
cort
of ar
desc
Low
high
stud
diffe
put,
liftir
post
spor
(arg
elite
atter
those

A
Lind
from
Olyn
speci
categ
zone
or M
impo
headi
a san

W.D. Russell (2001) examined different quantitative and qualitative aspects of flow in 42 elite athletes recruited from different team and individual sports and obtained a result almost completely in agreement with the nine identified components with regard to factors contributing to the zone experience. However, Russell considered the situation incomplete unless one took into consideration the dimensions that hindered or disturbed flow. In other words, those day to day occupational factors that we allow to break our concentration and focus.

Jackson (1995) has suggested that factors disturbing or disrupting zone in athletes and warriors be considered more or less uncontrollable, at least the external ones. One such important basic factor is "physical and mental readiness" (Jackson, 1992), which is necessary for the coordination of all perceptual-based decisions and subsequent movements, thus also a necessity for flow and zone. This factor is also a condition for action and awareness to create a context thereby in line with the second factor. "Physical and mental readiness" may be interpreted as mind and body coordination to achieve timing of activity (e.g., Benvenuti, Stanhope, Thomas, Panzer and Hallet, 1997; Hase & Stein, 1999; Strauss & Klich, 1999). Studies within this area point to the obligation of considering the gender variable whereby gender differences may underlie intensity and velocity of movement (Buchman, Leurgans, Gottlieb, Chen, Almeida and Corcos, 2000).

Technical skill affects both timing and muscle tension. Aggelousis, et al (2001) performed a study involving 41 subjects, aged 19–26 years, who were required to develop a new way of throwing a ball. Analysis of four muscles in the elbow region showed that conditions allowing more training gave better performance accompanied by reduced tension in the agonist muscle and in the most important antagonist muscle. These results confirmed those of an earlier study (Engelhorn, 1988) done with children aged 7-11 where performance enhancement through exercise was associated with reduced activity in the muscles analyzed.

The power of psychological variables on timing and muscle tension has been subjected to investigation (e.g., Braathen &

Svebak, 1990) that indicated that the effects of frustration (Rychtecky, 1978), anxiety and worry (Adam & van Wieringen, 1988) enhances or aggravates tension, while deep relaxation (Norlander, Bergman & Archer, 1999), visualization (Harris & Robinson, 1986) and self-talk (Harris & Robinson, 1986) reduces tension and mitigate aggravation. Bird (1987) described an experimental case-study where an elite level 23-year-old rifle marksman demonstrated that the most successful performance was associated with ability to attain relatively low levels of cortical activation. Between "taking-aim" and "firing," his level of anxiety remained stable until an instant before firing, when it descended sharply, rising again to normal level after firing. Lower levels of anxiety during a series were associated with higher scores. Further, Janson (1995) reported a series of case-studies indicating that the most successful athletes within different disciplines (i.e., bowling, boxing, archery, discus, shot-put, hammer, javelin, cycling, golf, marksmanship and weight-lifting) often produced lower anxiety levels, pre-, during- and post-action, than less successful athletes, in each respective sport: this finding was confirmed even in the case of boxing (arguably a technical activity). Janson (1995) noted, too, that elite athletes show a markedly higher degree of synchronized attendance to arousal and anxiety to a much greater extent than those less skillful.

A series of tests and studies were done by Norlander, Gård, Lindholm & Archer, in 2003, by interacting with elite athletes from a wide variety of disciplines and skill levels, including Olympic level athletes. 33 specific categories were created and specific performances and experiences were related to each of the categories. The 33 categories were derived from an analysis of zone and flow. A numeric scoring system of **Meaningful Units**, or **MUs**, was assigned to each category to determine its level of importance or level of experience. Under each respective category heading is a short explanation of the category, and is followed by a sampling of commentary from the test subjects.

Results

1. **When timing happens everything seems to fit. (106 MUs)**
    All aspects of co-ordination must fit in motion, thought and time exactly when one is about to perform a task.

Examples:

- "Timing is for me when everything fits without having to think about it"
- "It is much easier to perform good results if my timing is right"
- "An unbelievably concentrated and tough job facilitates timing completely, it's just there even if I feel exhausted and have pains"

2. **Concentration is the most important psychological factor. (86 MUs)**
    Concentration is described as an essential condition for performance. It is critical that individuals develop the ability to concentrate upon the right things prior to a difficult task.

Examples:

- "When I am concentrated days before an important event I have difficulty mixing with outside activities"
- "I can never have good timing without having good concentration at the same time"
- "All interfering thoughts must be removed. Those I must avoid. It is the performance that is important"

3. **Preparation and warm-up is highly important. (77 MUs)**
    The basis for a good result is that one is very well prepared through well-planned and hard training. In this way thoughts directed towards what will happen for a long time.

Examples:

- "The brain controls the body. That is what I train for a long time. Already at the start of the season I mark the most important events. If something specific is the goal I train and adjust the brain upon that high demand event"
- "I must have everything prepared before an event, nothing must be left to chance. I must have control of everything"
- "Sitting down and thinking too much before the start soon feels bad. What one has to do one has done many times before. I have my plan and I know how I shall carry out the event"

4.   **Develop methods for tackling problematic high demand situations. (54 MUs)**
     Many situations and disturbances, amongst others, one's own negative thoughts, may burden individuals in the process of performing at level competition. There are many ways by which one may solve difficulties before and during an event.

Examples:

- "If I am tired, for example, due to a long travel or bad sleep before an event, I must mobilize my inner reverses"
- "I usually divide up the event into different parts and teach myself during training how I shall deal with tactical aspects, for example, what to do at the start, in the middle or at the end"
- "I can accept being beaten if I have performed well. The quality of the competition is higher if many are in good form, but it is more difficult to win"

5.   **This is how I want to feel in high demand events. (47 MUs)**
     Often it is positive to feel in good form. But there are individuals who perform maximally despite not experiencing the feeling of being in top form.

Examples:

- "It is a good test already at the start of an event if I'm in good form, whether the equipment works, how I perform on this arena, how the wind is blowing, if everything is working it is a wonderful feeling"
- "If I have good rhythm which is important for me, I can await breaks in the wind"
- "At the end of the event, I count down and try to focus, coupling in the autopilot"

6. **The training schedule and plan are critical for a good result. (46 MUs)**

   It is very clear how important it is to have a very good training lay-out, planning and thoroughly thought-out strategies. In younger, less experienced individuals, discipline, with regard to development of technique, is very important, whereas veterans alter their training to suit the conditions.

Examples:

- "Once I trained on unbroken terrain at maximum speed, up and down hills, through moss, I just rushed forward, in this case it was more about training of attitude than about the speed of getting me forward"
- "If I feel that it's heavy going, I still give maximum effort. Tough going is no obstacle to hard training"
- "In my sport, there was earlier more amount of training compared with now, when one focuses on qualitative training"

7. **One must be prepared for problems. (45 MUs)**

   Individuals are often confronted by difficult mental/physical situations, e.g. tiredness. Thus, it is necessary that they are prepared for when these situations arise and have the right strategies for dealing with the problem.

Examples:

- "One must be prepared for problems at significant event, for example the equipment had technical problems"

- "If I feel resistance from my body, it's wrong now you must rest now, then I break off training instead of continuing for two hours"
- "There are always small failures; it is nothing that one can influence oneself"

8. **Control should encompass preparations and situations around the event, never in the execution itself or in the technical details. (42 MUs)**
   Everyone answers that they want control over what happens around training and the competition. But none want to have conscious control of details in their technical execution.

Examples:

- "Control is something positive for me, what I get up in my head is that I shall have control over preparations before the event"
- "Control is quite important for me; I'm a control-freak who commands the situation. The equipment must be 'tip-top' and everything around must be under my control, as much as necessary for an important competition, then it feels good"
- "If I have bad control of any part it'll go badly, I can never shirk with that, then it gets discovered"

9. **Mental training is carried out according to one's own models. (40 MUs)**
   All of the individuals applied mental training, but have developed their own models that they have placed complete trust in

Examples:

- "I prepare myself mentally before an event through successive mental repetitions of what I need to do 'when-the-chips-are-down'"
- "With regard to the mental training one must think right, normally there's not much disturbance, but training mentally when alone is better, it feels good"

- "Many technical details are part of mental preparation. That is what one looks for in the training of timing"

10. **Mental steps in important competitions. (40 MUs)**
    Thoughts may run away down a path counterproductive for performance. It is essential to return to the right mental outlook if thoughts are astray

Examples:

- "I usually think of a computer that has control/alt/delete, if I press these tangents the screen will be black, it's a good image for 'zero-position, after that I load what's there"
- "Sometimes I'm on the borderline of making a bad result, but it works out anyway, then I smile to myself and confess I've been lucky"
- "If I'm behind then there's a fight within me to produce what is necessary"

11. **Nervousness before and during an important event exists even for the most successful. That type of stress may influence the result in a positive direction. (40 MUs)**
    Despite great arousal and anxiety, those at the top still manage to give top performances when it's necessary. The consensus is that one is extremely nervous before, and sometimes during, the competitions, but one succeeds very well anyway.

Examples:

- "Long before the event I was very nervous and went around worrying but after the event, it was hard to understand why I was so nervous"
- "I know that when I've got a bit into the event I'm so nervous that it feels bad, but it works anyway"
- "Nervousness and fear of failure are feelings within me"

12. **Bad timing can occur. (40 MUs)**
    Even if it works well before the event, can timing be disrupted when most necessary?

Examples:

- "I must really exert myself if it's a day when my timing is only half-way good"
- "If timing is working badly I must take emergency measures"
- "If things are going badly I have to find my timing again, but it can be difficult"
- "In order to break a bad trend one has to be absolutely professional"

13. **It is important to have a knowledgeable and understanding coach. (35 MUs)**
     If one is to have a trainer he has to be of absolute top class; otherwise it is just as well to be without one.

Examples:

- "Once my trainer asked me to go and see him, 'had I fooled around or …?' instead he said that he believed in me and that I ought to train my technique, if I did that I would be above expectation, someone believed in me and was proven correct"
- "Perhaps one doesn't think about it when one is standing there, but as a trainer I think one has to consider all the bits as a whole"
- "My trainer has had great significance for my timing, I had to begin by learning the movements in slow motion"

14. **It is important to get the right feeling. (29 MUs)**
     Feeling is part of that 'wholeness' that is experienced as the basis of performance and the way to achieve good timing.

Examples:

- "One is charged with feeling somewhere"
- "Right feeling involves only the mental"
- "I've often started competing too early, tired myself out in the competition before it's even begun, it's necessary to have the right balance emotionally"

15. **This is my way to carry out a competition. (21 MUs)**
Obviously, before an important event the ways in which one prepares varies greatly. Each has his/her own way to 'pep up' or view different situations.

Examples:

- "I never think that I shall win, never at all, I do my best and try to get to the final, anything longer I never think of"
- "I did the wrong things completely in the beginning of my career; it was a difficult lesson that had to be relearned"
- "I took a break of two years from competition and then came back. During the break I was able to consider what I had done during the earlier years. After my 'come-back' I would give particular thought to execution before a competition"

16. **To a great extent, training ought to be like the competition. (21 MUs)**
The best, further forward in their careers, will carry out quality training that mimics realistic conditions as much as possible.

Examples:

- "I find it quite easy to envision myself into real-world situations during training"
- "At training I want to create an experience of the body, feeling that anxiety one gets at important times and then succeed with what I have set myself"
- "I trained with the best in the world; that was very good"

17. **More radical technique alterations should be carried out in younger years. (21 MUs)**
If more radical adjustments of technique are required; these should be done in younger years. But lesser adjustments, improvements and developments are maintained continually within the elite group.

Examples:

- "I have developed the whole time during my career and I have discovered small improvements the whole time"
- "I have developed my technique myself; no one has meant anything for me in that regard"
- "Technique adjustments are made during training, never at competition"

18. **Visualization is applied to arrive at the right feeling/flow before and during performance. (19 MUs)**

Examples:

- "It is my 'driving-thought' that steers everything"
- "Visualization is about how I fantasize about how concordant it should be in relation to the goal, OK, this is how, now to the next thing"
- "If I have difficulties envisioning the goal, I perform badly"

19. **Self-confidence is an important basis for good performance. (19 MUs)**
    Self-confidence is a psychological factor that improves through training and achievement. It is further developed by having knowledge that others view our performance, skills and abilities in a positive way.

Examples:

- "If I don't believe in myself I am hardly likely to attain timing either"
- "Good timing is good and I have good self-confidence and if self-confidence is bad then timing is bad, too"
- "My self-confidence hangs together with good self-confidence"

20. **Execution is taken care of unconsciously. (16 MUs)**
    This is a part of performance, difficult to explain and difficult to understand, that one may perform so many tasks unconsciously and without having complete control over what is happening.

Examples:

- "I think the brain sees the goal but is not able to register it consciously (a very fast-moving activity)"
- "I use one or two words to engage the autopilot and that great feeling I want in the technique"
- "I can perform well without seeing the goal"

21. **The atmosphere within the whole team is important. (15 MUs)**

The team members and leaders ought to best understand what must be done and what services each individual requires to optimize performance. It seems likely that a sufficient degree of 'pep-talk' from colleagues is more valuable than that of others.

Examples:

- "The team is working badly if one thinks ill of certain persons' behavior"
- "Co-ordination within the team works even if one was competing singly, there are those who want to join closer to the competition, let them do so"
- "One agrees with the leader and the athlete how it should be done."

22. **Inspiration from the task is important for achieving a good result. (13 MUs)**

The consensus is that inspiration from the task is another factor contributing to top performance.

Examples:

- "One can hardly be 100% inspired at a small competition even if I've tried to get a good result. It can feel heavy sometimes at small competitions"
- "Inspiration must be present at training and competition to make it meaningful; what I do is important"
- "Inspiration is there the whole time, for me it's a question of attaining the right offensive puzzle bits that I want to think about"

23. **Technique is well-rehearsed and works automatically in competitions where everything goes well. (13 MUs)**
    The better the active athletes have become the fewer changes in technique that have been made.

Examples:

- "The technique has become part of me and my behavior that has been ingrained over a very long period and is difficult to alter"
- "I am very careful that the technique is executed exactly as rehearsed"
- "The technique is in my backbone; it very easy to compete when everything works"

24. **I have not received any good coaching. (11 MUs)**
    Several of the athletes have not had a regular coach. One is autodidactic to a very great extent.

Examples:

- "I went through the whole junior stage completely with my own resources only"
- "I am self-taught"
- "No coach can come to me and say, this is what you do today"

25. **Motivation and attitude influence the will to train hard and compete. (11 MUs)**
    Motivation appears to be so obvious a factor for most individuals they don't even mention it.

Examples:

- "Motivation is important"
- "I must have a competitive consciousness that carries me through the tough 'building-up' training"
- "Others have said to me, 'What are you doing?' I must have something that drives me forward"

26.   **Negative thoughts are to be avoided. (11 MUs)**
      Without forethought, unwished-for thoughts may 'pop-up'
      like a 'jack-in-the-box'

Examples:

- "Thoughts can give a whole lot of problems"
- "During major events I have tried to steer my thoughts away
  from negative thinking"
- "The thought can do something so that I become heavy in my
  movements"

27.   **Sometimes one must alter thinking to seek good
      timing. (9 MUs)**
      In order to seek a way into good timing one must act.

Examples:

- "If I make several mistakes I can try and alter my thoughts,
  hardly after just a single mistake"
- "I alter thoughts easily in order to get into good timing"
- "When I seek good timing I change thoughts absolutely"

28.   **The translation of timing in the dictionary is com-
      pletely correct. (9 MUs)**
      The English "Timing" translates to time-adjustment, adap-
      tation, adjustment and regulating.

Examples:

- "The definition fits exactly for me"
- "The definitions in the dictionary apply for me, it is a con-
  firmation that I am right, it's good to know"
- "I can relate completely to the definitions"

29.   **In a competition thoughts must be strategic or not
      at all. (8 MUs)**
      It appears to be important to consider the whole event
      rather than details in order to get technical aspects to
      work.

Examples:

- "The more tired I am the shorter my planning. I just think fighting-to-the-last-drop"
- "I need to have a thought strategy: I'll do my best"
- "In the physical part of my sport I don't want to think of anything at all."

30. **When everything works well all movements are smooth. (6 MUs)**
    Within sport, when one refers to"smoothness" one implies that it is easy to execute the task and that one has less need for conscious thinking and steering of one's action. Most aspects "run" by themselves and have luck on one's side.

Examples:

- "At the Olympics it was rigid at first, then later everything just worked"
- "The best is when the competition just happens, then there is no time to think about anything but the competition"
- "I try to avoid looking for problems and instead focus myself to try and find automatic executions again"

31. **Timing can 'come-and-go.' (5 MUs)**
    If one loses timing it can be difficult, but not impossible, to rediscover it again.

Examples:

- "If I become tired I can lose my timing"
- "On a certain rare occasion during a competition, one could awake suddenly and 'pick-up' good timing"
- "I have never succeeded in executing a whole competition in which I retained that 'bubble-dream', for sooner or later it bursts, and unwelcome thoughts come in and then one reacts so that timing operates badly"

32. **One must act in the right way if technique starts to be disrupted. (5 MUs)**

    If one encounters a state in which technique is disturbed it is essential that the individual concerned returns to basic technique and in this way eventually corrects the deviation that may have occurred to 'competitive-stress'.

Examples:

- "Even if technique is working badly at a competition I never ruin everything, something works, but it was something else that happened"
- "If I've been in training where I come home well-trained but with slightly worse technique that was corrected by my trainer"
- "One lane can work well, whereas another not at all, everything can go wrong."

33. **Thought, image and feeling should work together. (4 MUs)**

Examples:

- "The total co-ordination is important"
- "Thought, image and feeling should all be present if good timing is to be achieved"
- "All three functions have importance for me."

All the participants in the study reported the necessity of maintaining the right "basic thoughts" when they were trying to perform at their absolute best. The following diagram depicts the culmination of how the participants in the above study saw their drive and how correct timing was achieved for maximum performance.

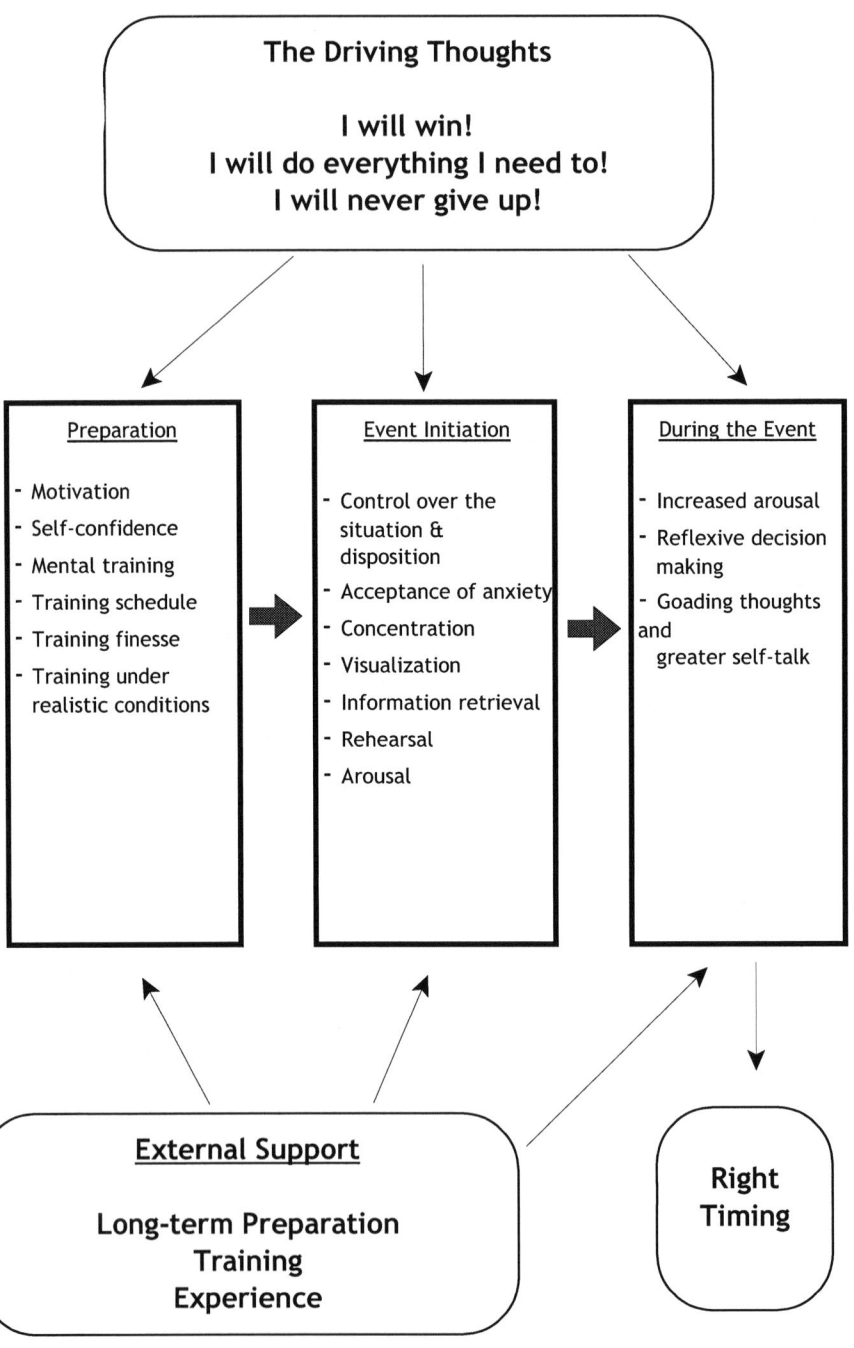

The study results from the 33 categories were formed into six main groups, or themes. This was done through independent reflections by each of the researchers. The **first theme** indicates that there is a **unifying "driving" thought** that propels the top level athletes and warriors towards their goal. The **second theme** describes the preparations that pass by the major task. The **third theme** describes how one has executed the final preparations, just prior to the start of an event. The **fourth theme** explains how one has experienced the execution of the event. The **fifth theme** describes something about how the individual experienced the support that they received. As a product of these five themes, the achievement of good timing during performance presents itself for the participants: this is the **sixth theme.**

The **first theme** covers two categories, according to the previous results section (18 and 29). These categories may be described as a **"driving thought,"** a form of trigger that through its force drives the warrior towards his or her goal. It can be described as the will to win and it is generally very strong. Thoughts like **"I'll do it all"** indicate that these warriors possess a great 'driving-force' that implements their victories. Under the categories 2, 3 and 4, the driving thought is always present, like a background sound, as one participant expressed it: "Somewhere in the brain the thought 'I shall do my best' always exists." In theme 3, the athletes describe how they reinforce the overriding thought through conscious, decisive and recurrent thinking about the "driving thought."

The **second theme** covers 8 categories (numbers: 3, 4, 6, 9, 16, 17, 19 and 25) that deal with the **long-term preparation** before important events. There exists a vast amount of training invested by each of the male and female participants in the study. The extent of this preparatory work is described in the second theme by different categories. Physiological and psychological factors are noted both separately and in combination. These include motivation, self-confidence, and nervousness prior to high demand events, mental training, the format of training, technical finesse, training under real-world conditions and preparations. The "driving thought" provides the necessary motivation which is the fundamental requirement for warriors to train as hard as is demanded. This level of motivation is so strong that the warrior will typically commit to greater exertion, despite the time already spent and the pain experienced. The other categories within this theme are highly dependent upon motivation. All the factors comprising this theme pertain to the individual's way of training and coping with the pressures that elite level events exert upon the absolute best warriors.

The **third theme** covered 6 categories (2, 8, 11, 14, 22, and 26) that may be summarized as the **direct mental preparation prior to the start of an event**. Several of the participants consider it very important that their thoughts are strategically oriented and most speak of **envisioning** what they expect will happen. In this circumstance, it must be noted that concentration was considered the most essential psychological factor. This illustrates that individuals need absolute solitude, away from media, managers, trainers and other acquaintances that may make the wrong comments at that time. Concentration may be interpreted in several ways, from "narrow focus" to "split vision," depending upon the particular task at hand. Mobilizing the "right" concentration ensures, too, that negative thoughts are kept aside and unity with the "driving thought" is reinforced (theme 1). All the participants described the necessity of "concentration exercise" as critical, just prior to and during an event, a procedure used to project an image of execution and/or accomplishment. The most desirable concentration is that with narrow focus, one that implies the absorption into oneself, **internal concentration**. This type of focus realizes a **scanning** of their bodies (the feeling of right level of tension), accomplishes a mental **retrieval** of correct execution, and reminds them that they possess the right technique and abilities within themselves. Concurrently, one repeats mentally the sequences inherent to the event, **rehearsal**, and the feeling so induced is essential for self-sufficiency just before start, a prerequisite for the desired **arousal or priming**.

Some of the participants in the study expressed a feeling of weakness just before the initiation of an event, but nevertheless recover their ability when the competition has started, as these feelings can facilitate priming or reaching the required level of arousal. Some form of "fighting-spirit" is generated as the event starts and this in turn initiates the technical ability. The awareness that they can perform well, despite the discomforts prior to initiation, generating this "fighting-spirit." All detailed thoughts regarding technique and accomplishment must be abandoned just before start, placing more emphasis on process rather than outcome.

All the participants sought control over situational aspects of the events, i.e. schedules, training and supervisory departures, start-times, etc. Possessing more comprehensive control over the situation is considered to optimize the possibility of better timing. In a different situation, Mack (1995) describes the importance, under emergency, of professions like law enforcement, military and firefighters possessing knowledge of events. Possession of information concerning how things look on the ground, what has occurred and prevailing conditions, were ranked highest and it was concluded that knowledge of what will happen allows mental preparation and ensures a substantially better job (Mack, 1995).

The **fourth theme** covers 10 categories (5, 7, 10, 12, 20, 23, 27, 30, 31 and 32) that describe the participants' **experiences during performance**. It is now when one needs good timing. If the component parts of the third theme work effectively, most individuals assume that they achieve increased potential to realize a natural feeling of zone and flow (Jackson & Csikszentmihályi, 2000). However, not all warriors since the present ones implied that one may feel heavy and stiff before start and they could experience a great load, psychological and physical, during the initial stage of an event. Despite these wearing periods, often throughout an event, it is remarkable that the event is completed in the manner one applies. Normally, some sort of avoidance may be expected, breaking off or reducing the demands on oneself and performing worse. Top elite athletes seem to possess a strong 'winner-instinct' or 'driving-thought' that despite all setbacks during preparation and performance accept the discomforts to achieve the goal. Good timing may occur despite the 'heavy' feeling before or during an event: "Timing can come or go," related one of the participants. A characteristic feature of the absolute best is that they never give up.

When thoughts, images, feelings and actions form a unity, one approaches the term timing. Perfect timing may be attained even under great stress or pressure and thinking constraints regarding risk of failure. The participants implied that even under these circumstances a good result may be achieved. One may attain good timing when under tough psychological pressure and thereby perform well.

The **fifth theme** covers 4 categories (13, 15, 21 and 24) and concerns the **training, supervising and external support** that the participants had received. On one hand, this part enters generally long before the warrior is called into performance. On the other, it concerns the final preparations before event initiation and for some of them, even during an event, through efforts of trainers and others. Team spirit appears as an important factor for peak performance, as external support was critical for several.

The **sixth theme, timing** (Categories 1, 28 and 33), emerges for the warriors if the five preceding themes can provide a functional basis. Category 1 provided the most MUs, 106, which is understandable since the study involved timing. Despite the variety of responses with a range of individual variations it is remarkable that the subjects' responses display such agreement over what the concept entails, i.e. temporal setting, adaptation, adjustment and regulation.

Characteristics of Zone and Flow

Now, having identified, or at least discussed, factors that contribute or are experienced by the elite when functioning in the zone, let's delve a little further as to what the zone is, its relevance to the realm of the warrior and what a warrior might feel in the zone.

Psychologists and peak performance trainers are continuously seeking cutting edge methods of achieving the most expedient route to establish true confidence, the trust in one's ability, appropriate focus, composure and explosive power with graceful, efficient patterns of movement. This is characteristic of almost all high level performance, including team and individual pursuits, both are rewarded when flowing, powerful movements can be performed with effortless composure.

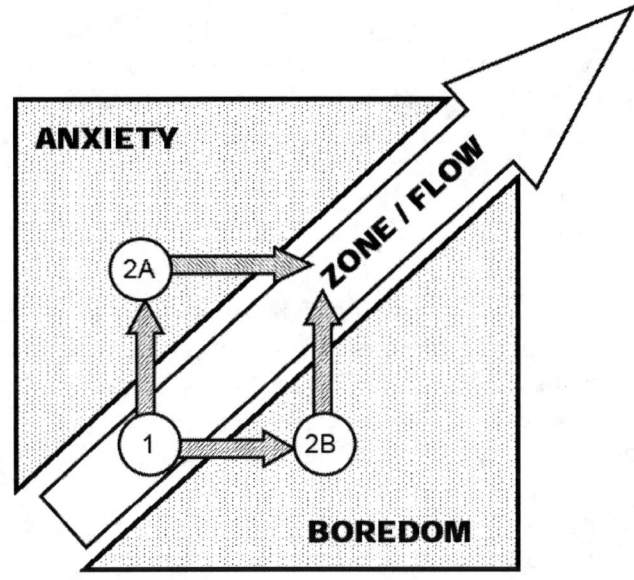

THE WARRIOR (1) WILL MOVE OUT OF FLOW AND BECOME BORED. AS HIS SKILL IN AN ACTIVITY INCREASES (2A), UNLESS THE CHALLENGE TO SUCCEED ALSO INCREASES, LIKEWISE, A WARRIOR (1) WILL MOVE OUT OF FLOW IF THE DEMAND ON HIM IS TOO GREAT (2B) TO STAY IN FLOW, HE MUST INCREASE HIS LEVEL OF SKILL.

The following are the various characteristics of **zone**:

1. Relaxed

Not psyched up. Research has consistently shown the best performance occurs when an individual is just slightly above their normal state of arousal, not at the far end of the spectrum as once thought. Energized, yet relaxed, a balance of quiet intensity.

2. Confident

Not allowing a lapse in performance to undermine belief in ability. When you perform well, you feel confident regardless of the odds, knowing you will be on top. The warrior exudes confidence, pride and discipline. Confidence on the inside is outwardly expressed by individual presence, walk and facial expressions. The warrior should always expect to succeed, not hope or wish to.

3. Focused

The warrior is completely absorbed in the moment. No memory of the past and no issues about the future; the warrior is here and now! Concentrating only on the mission at hand. Oblivious to everything else going on around him or her and consumed by the moment with no sense of time.

4. Instinctive

No interference from thought or emotion. Things happen without contest and without active consent, as if on "auto pilot." The body just seems to know what to do without conscious directive.

5. Effortless

All moves are smooth, purposeful and on time. The individual is in a state of mind and body where great things can happen with little effort. The mind and the body are working with one another in perfect unison.

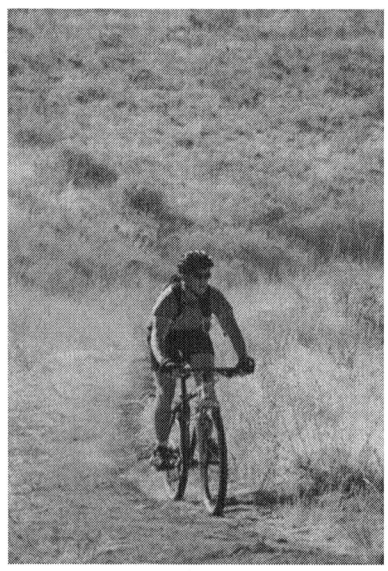

The phenomenon of zone or flow is most commonly associated with elite athletes, but can be a valuable state for individuals in any high demand situation.

6. Fun

Oh yes, fun! As counter-politically correct as it may be to discuss fun in the same conversation as preparation for conflict, the enjoyment felt when in the zone is like none other. Comparable to feeling like a child enjoying a game with pure and innocent delight. Because of this, fun is a key aspect of emotion control under stress.

7. Control

The warrior is in control! What he thinks and what he wants to happen will! The warrior is in ultimate command of senses and emotions—controlling them, not the other way around. When you are in control, you are in charge.

Success in conflict requires the mind and the body together. Take some time and consider some past peak and near peak performances; it can be a great aid setting the tone for the future.

Confidence

Confidence is a state of mind commonly linked to success. The importance of high levels of confidence in warriors is highlighted in the studies of Jones and Hardy (1990) and Henry (1986). Jones and Hardy's report, based on the experiences of elite athletes, not million-dollar free-agent athletes who get into fist fights with fans and push rap albums harder than they play their sport, but honest to goodness high performance elite athletes, like the ones who run marathons, expedition races, and win Olympic gold. The study found that, in general, individuals tended to have extreme levels of confidence and felt that their levels were needed for a desired level of performance. Henry's study of elite athletes showed that 90% of those interviewed had high levels of self-confidence (Henry 1986).

Confidence is usually a result of an individual anticipating success in a pending event. An individual's anticipated outcome is the greatest indicator of confidence (Kaues 1980). The expectation of success can be based on an individual's confidence in themselves, teammates, goals, strategies, physical condition, or in the trainer (Kaues 1980).

Elite athletes are well-known for their high levels of confidence, well, at least the successful ones. It is believed that this is likely a result of being an elite athlete and not necessarily a cause, something like a "by-product," "confidence levels mirror skill level" (DeVenzio 1997). This specific view points to the link between talent or previous success and confidence levels. If this is true, then quite likely the best remedy for low confidence is success. Coaches and trainers in all pursuits have used this tactic for as long as competitive events have existed; it's often used when coaches or athletic director's schedule games against lower ranked teams, so that they can rack up wins and boost confidence.

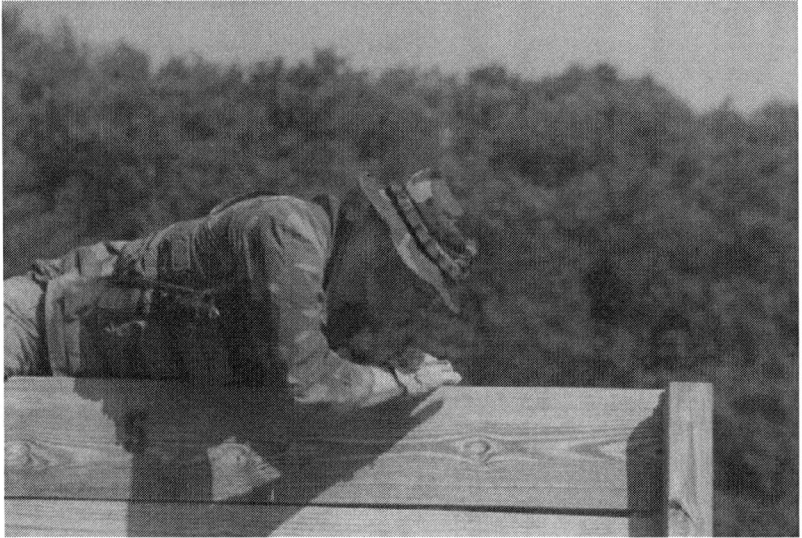

Elite athletes and warriors alike are well-known for their high levels of confidence, a by-product of an expectation of success in a situation.

I believe that one cannot clearly define confidence as a cause or effect of being elite. It is obvious that to reach the very pinnacle of performance, an individual must have a high level of confidence in their abilities; and getting to that elite level, and all preceding successes that it took to get to that level, must build the confidence level of an individual.

Anxiety

The link between anxiety and performance in high demand pursuits has been known for a long time. Stories abound of individuals and organizations that performed poorly because they underestimated their opponent or worried themselves out of a situation. Dealing with anxiety successfully is an important characteristic of a warrior.

Research has shown that the ability to cope with pressure and anxiety is an integral part of high demand activities, particularly among the elite (Hardy et al. 1996; Orlick & Partington 1988). One of the earliest models that attempted to explain the relationship between arousal/anxiety and performance was the inverted-U hypothesis: it stated that as arousal increased so would performance; but if arousal became too great, performance would deteriorate. In other words, as stress began to build and an individual still felt confident in their ability to control it, performance would improve. However, once the stress became so great, at a level that the individual perceived it as uncontrollable and started doubting their ability to manage it, performance would decline rapidly.

An individualistic approach was added to this hypothesis when researchers developed the concept of *individualized zones of optimal functioning* or IZOFs (Hanin 1980, 1986). According to this theory, each individual has an optimal level of performance anxiety. If the individual is in the "zone," peak performance will be the result. However, if anxiety levels are too high or too low, optimum results will not be achieved (Hanin 1980, 1986). IZOFs can be determined by repeatedly measuring anxiety and performance or through an individual's recall of anxiety during performance.

Clearly, anxiety levels can have a variety of effects on performance. These effects vary based on the anxiety and on the individual. Fortunately, research has shown anxiety can be reduced through training, experience, mental imagery and cognitive intervention (Meyers et al. 1982; Holm et al. 1996). These methods not only aim at reducing stress and anxiety levels, but also to improve confidence levels and enhance mechanical skills. The goal is to help the warrior to enter his or her IZOF.

Personally, I think that confidence levels and anxiety are closely related. The higher an individual's confidence, the less he or she will worry about conflict and outcome, they know they are prepared and ready. Likewise, if an individual is over-anxious, it may be a sign of self-doubt.

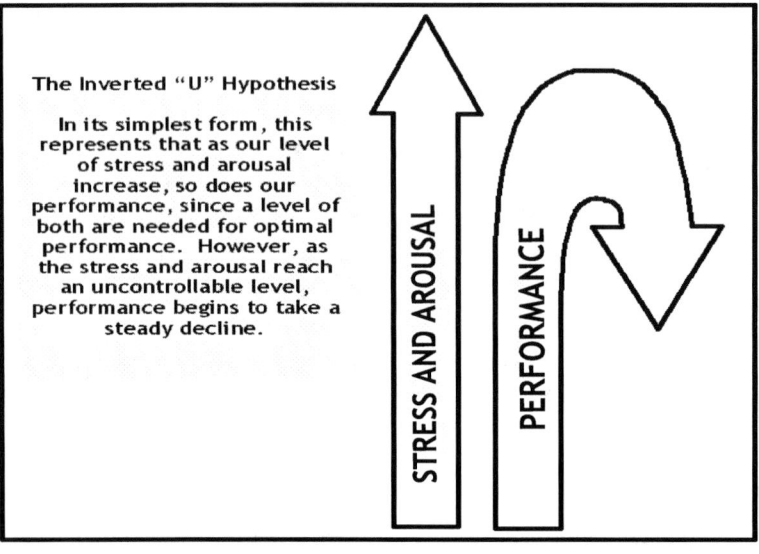

The Inverted "U" Hypothesis

In its simplest form, this represents that as our level of stress and arousal increase, so does our performance, since a level of both are needed for optimal performance. However, as the stress and arousal reach an uncontrollable level, performance begins to take a steady decline.

STRESS AND AROUSAL

PERFORMANCE

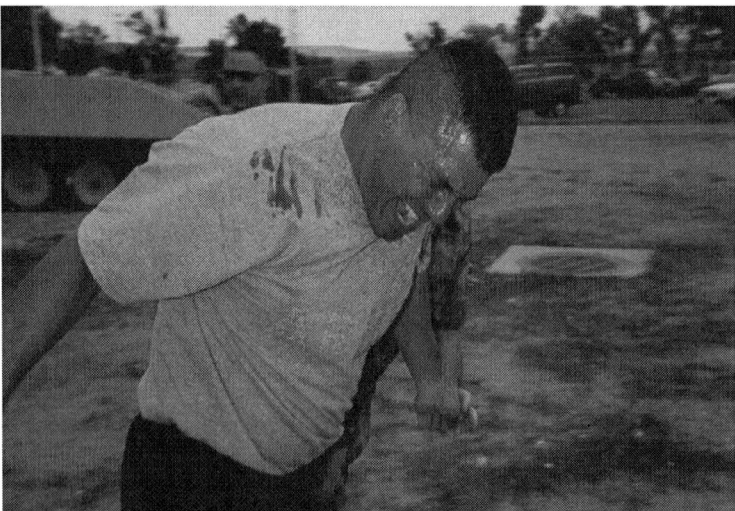

Anxiety levels can have a variety of effects on performance. These effects vary based on the anxiety, the individual and the individual's prior training, conditioning and experience.

Pre-competitive Anxiety

Imagine that it is the day before a large planned operation and the warrior begins to worry about how well he or she will perform. The individual may find that worrying begins to feed on itself, creating further areas of concern that were not previously considered. This is a simple example of *pre-competitive anxiety* (PCA), one of the most debilitating variables in performance, especially under high stress and high demand situations.

Pre-competitive anxiety is a state of arousal that is unpleasant, negative and destructive, typically occurring within the 24-hour time span prior to a specific and expected event. The worry that is associated with PCA is not just experienced with our heads, but with our entire body. Our bodies provide us with numerous cues such as muscle tension, butterflies, frequent compulsion to urinate and cotton mouth and suggests that we are out of control. Thoughts become self-focused, self-defeating and negative. Most individuals experience a combination of these responses during a pre-event period. However, the degree to which they influence our performance is heavily dependent on the interaction of our own uniqueness and with the situation. In other words, it is based on the level of our training, conditioning and experiences.

The Sources of PCA

Pre-competitive anxiety results from an imbalance between perceived capabilities and the demands of the situation and environment. When the perceived demands are balanced by the perceived capabilities, the warrior is getting ready to experience optimal arousal. This is what I refer to throughout this manual as zone or flow state. In this state, everything appears to go smoothly, almost effortlessly. However, if your perceived capabilities exceed the challenge, arousal will decrease, resulting in boredom or lack of motivation, If the opposite occurs (perceived challenges exceed capabilities), you will become overly aroused, resulting in worry and anxiety. As you can assume, PCA results when skills and abilities are not perceived as equivalent to the challenge. Research by Walter Kroll demonstrated that at least five specific factors trigger PCA:

1. *Physical complaints*—digestive disturbances, shaking and yawning.

2. *Fear of failure*—losing, choking, living up to expectations, and making mistakes.

3. *Feelings of inadequacy*—unprepared, poor conditioning, low skill/ability, and feelings that something is wrong.

4. *Loss of control*—being jinxed, bad luck, poor planning, and inclement weather.

5. *Guilt*—concerns about hurting an opponent, fear of getting in trouble, and cheating.

Whether or not you experience PCA is dependent upon several other factors, such as skill level, experience, and your general level of arousal in daily activities.

How PCA Affects Performance

There are two primary ways that PCA can affect a warrior's performance.

First, a high state of physical arousal may be counter-productive to a specific activity. For situations requiring endurance, power, or both, PCA can be very draining on a warrior's energy level. In situations where calmness is critical (e.g., dedicated marksman, negotiations, planning), PCA can significantly interfere with your ability to stay calm. A high state of physical arousal can also interfere with situations requiring a focused channeling of power. Effective performances in these situations require some muscles to be tense and others to be relaxed. Overly tense muscles ineffectively transfer their power. The increased tension usually interferes with this channeling. Examples of such events include hitting with a baton, kicking or punching, and field events such as running in a foot pursuit.

Second, research has demonstrated that anxiety can significantly interfere with your ability to think clearly. When you are anxious, your thoughts generally turn inward to focus on yourself, which may result in an inappropriate focusing of attention. Actions that were once automatic require constant, often competing thought, which further interferes with your ability to adjust to make quick, on-the-spot decisions. In addition, these thoughts may be negative and result in preoccupation with what you can't do, rather than what you can do.

Does Nervousness Always Mean Bad Performance?

Definitely not! Whenever you anticipate an event that is important to you, it is normal to feel some nervousness. In fact, it is a sign of readiness. This type of readiness is known as positive arousal and is usually referring to many of the physical cues you experience. Elite warriors channel this energy to work for them rather than against them. Answers to the following questions may help you distinguish between positive arousal and negative anxiety:

1. How much does my endeavor require me to be psyched up as I enter the situation? Some situations may require a higher state of arousal (e.g., building search) than others (e.g., crime scene preservation).

2. Do I often have thoughts of self-doubt about my ability?

3. Do I often have thoughts about factors that are beyond my control?

Answering "Yes" to the last two questions is an indication that the individual is moving from positive arousal to negative anxiety. If you find yourself nervous but still confident in your ability, that is a sign of readiness. However, worrying about your ability to perform at levels that you normally are able to perform with ease, or worrying about factors over which you have no control may interfere with your ability to enter an event mentally ready.

Recommendations for Warriors

1. *Become more aware of your optimal level of arousal.*

> Think of the times when you felt ready going into an event
> and it worked for you. Think of other times when you
> were anxious and it interfered with your performance.
> Being as specific as possible, write down the differences
> between these times based on three questions.
>
> - What thoughts made you feel ready, and what
>   thoughts made you anxious?
>
> - What feelings did you experience when you were ready
>   versus when you were anxious?
>
> - What were the differences in your behavior between
>   these times?

This will allow you to start looking for patterns that may help
you become more aware of what best prepares you mentally for
an event. Examples of when you were anxious may include
thinking about whether you had prepared enough for the
situation, exaggerating the skill of your opponent(s), or
exaggerating the importance of the outcome of the event.
Feelings may have been an overly high sense of arousal that led
you to emotionally "avoid" the event rather than "move toward"
the event. You may have found that, behaviorally, you were more
anxious when you were around others rather than by yourself.

The important point is to start understanding the factors that
allow you to become motivated, and the factors that tend to take
you too far. A good rule of thumb is to notice when you begin to
focus intently on the situation and become excited about
approaching the situation. This is a good indication that you are
reaching your optimal level, If self-doubt occurs and you are
having trouble putting it aside, you have most likely crossed into
the "anxiety zone." The following recommendations may help
during those times.

2. *Focus on things that are within your control.*

One of the major sources of anxiety is worrying about factors that are beyond your control. Your thoughts become preoccupied with a series of "what ifs." A great method of counter-balancing this attitude is to become more performance-oriented. Being performance-oriented means that you are concerned with the thing that is most in your control—your performance. Perform-ance-oriented warriors are more satisfied with a defeat if they performed their best, than if they had won and performed poorly. Conversely, being outcome-oriented means that you are concerned with one thing—the win. It doesn't matter how you get there, as long as you have the big "W." I am certainly not trying to suggest that winning is not important. It is crucial and it's the basis for this type of training. However, by placing the highest importance on the outcome, think of the added pressure you have placed upon yourself or your warriors.

We should hasten to add that it is unnecessary pressure. So many other factors beyond your control play into whether or not you win (e.g., the opponent's ability, where you are, your training, weather and other environmental conditions). Most of our anxiety lies in the fear of the unknown. We can reduce this fear by pulling in the ranks to focus on what is truly within our control. When you think about it, being more performance-oriented is likely to increase your chances of winning in a situation. You will be approaching the event focused on what you can do and what needs to be done to perform your best. In addition, as you begin concentrating on your performance in the pre-event period it is usually best to concentrate on your strengths. Focus on what you can do, not what you can't do. Practice is where you work on your weaknesses. The event is the time to capitalize on your strengths and on your improved areas. Therefore, focus intently on these areas.

If you feel your arousal level getting too high, take a moment to regroup and say to yourself, "OK, I'm going to show them what 1 can do, and not worry about what I can't do. I'm going to give 100% of the potential I have today." The bottom line is to learn to focus on doing the best you can with what you have at that moment, and view any positive outcome as a bonus. If you do well, take the time to focus on how that makes you feel. If you win, it makes your performance that much sweeter.

3. Use "performance cues" to develop or retrain your arousal level.

It is important to realize that with mental training you are developing skills in much the same way you develop physical and mechanical skills. You can recall when you were a rookie and first started learning a new level of your trade, how you had to think about every little detail. Eventually, as you practiced these new skills they became more habitual or reflexive. It is the same way with mental skills. Your typical arousal level has been developed over time and may have become habitual. To retrain your arousal level, you simply have to learn new mental routines and practice them until they become automatic. In critical situations, however, warriors may need to do this quickly, rather than constantly rehearse long statements to them. One helpful exercise is to reflect on how you want to perform given your present skill level. Your desired performance may be a collection of past accomplishments or an image of a future performance. Once you have a clear image of a desired performance, label that performance with a representative cue word, statement, or symbol. When doing this, you may choose to use a general cue that reflects your overall performance, or a cue that reflects a more specific part of your performance. In addition, you may want to incorporate a cue that reminds you of a time when you operated at your desired level.

Experiment with all three types of cues, separately or in combination, to determine which works best for you. The most important thing to remember is that this label must immediately recall the image of a performance that you want to create. An example is an officer who used the cue "explode" to represent explosive speed as a way of preparing for a combative suspect, and "hawk" to represent smooth graceful movements as a way of preparing for disciplined movement during a building search. The next step is incorporating this performance cue into your pre-event preparation (see chapter on self-talk). Reflect on your cue as a method of motivation. You can also use it to reduce your arousal level if you start experiencing anxiety. If you start feeling anxious, take a deep breath, relax, and repeat the cue to yourself. Try to focus fully on what it represents to you (see chapter on centering). This will result in bringing you back to performance-oriented thoughts that will properly prepare you for the competition.

With practice and repetition, these thoughts will become more habitual and capable of controlling your arousal level. The same principle is utilized often with music tapes. Many warriors have a favorite song that has the effect of psyching them up, and another song that relaxes them. During the pre-event period, they will listen to one or both of the songs at times when they want to modify their arousal levels. They have essentially found a performance cue that induces a feeling that they are trying to achieve. In the early 1980's, when I was fighting in full contact matches in Phoenix and Las Vegas, I would listen to Judas Priest's "You've Got Another Thing Comin' " to create this effect. The important thing is to find what's right for you. It may take some trial-and-error, but will eventually result in approaching an event in a manner that will allow you to enjoy your abilities at their optimal level.

Recommendations for Trainers

1. *Become aware of your own arousal levels and how they interact with the warrior and other trainers.*

It is important to spend time reflecting on your own arousal levels as a way of understanding how they impact your effectiveness in training and your impact on other's performances. Applying the suggestions in Recommendations for Warriors to your training performance can help you understand and develop your optimal arousal level, as well as deal with PCA.

2. *Understand your warriors, individually; how they react during a pre-event period.*

Recognize those warriors who are usually under-aroused and those who are usually over-aroused for the demands of the situation. The under-aroused warriors may be those who typically appear sluggish during the early parts of an event. The over-aroused warriors, on the other hand, can be detected most often by being strong "training-warriors." These are the warriors who do great in training but have trouble realizing their potential in real-world situations. Performances during real-world events are a regression for them rather than a progression.

3. *Allow time for warriors to individually prepare themselves mentally for an event.*

Research has demonstrated that the famous "win one for the gipper" pep-talks are relatively limited in their effectiveness. During pre-event preparation, it may be helpful to bring the team together to review and discuss strategy and goals. Following this meeting, individuals should be allowed some time on their own to prepare for the event in a way that is most effective for them. Do not underestimate the power of this gesture. Many warriors are very concerned about how they present themselves to their trainers or supervisors. If they have tapped into how you would like your warriors to prepare, they will most likely present that image to you. However, this may be totally opposite of what they need. Conveying the message that you respect their methods of preparation frees them up to devote time to it. Some warriors may want to be by themselves, some may want to prepare with others to discuss the pending event, and others may want to be with teammates for humorous small-talk as a way of reducing their anxiety. Some of my best jokes were told in the back of our team vehicle on the way to rip someone's front door off. Allow them to go through the trial-and-error of finding out what is best for them. Following this individual line, bring them back together and summarize the goals you hope to accomplish. In addition, incorporating individual time for the coaches is equally important for their preparation.

4. *Foster a performance-oriented attitude in your warriors.*

As was explained in Recommendations for Warriors, warriors need to focus on what they can control. So many factors beyond their control play a part as to whether they win. Placing a high priority on outcome results in unnecessary pressure and extra factors that warriors worry about.

Unfortunately, a trainer's and a leader's livelihood is dependent upon outcome. Job stability and opportunity for professional advancement usually hinges on the winning record. As stated before, we are not implying that winning is unimportant. I am stating, however, that placing winning as the top and sole priority can have negative effects on a warrior's mental preparation and subsequent performance. Remember, your greatest chance for a positive outcome is to have each warrior play at his or her potential.

This can best be achieved by having your warriors focus on what they can control in their performance. Teaching warriors to appreciate the importance of gauging success by how well they perform, according to their own potential rather than by other's standards, is one of the greatest lessons a trainer can teach.

5. *Be specific with your suggestions to help warriors with PCA.*

It is easy to create a situation where a warrior struggling with PCA starts to "worry about worrying." Be careful to keep helpful suggestions specific to the actions that the warrior finds troublesome, rather than identifying or characterizing the warrior by the weakness he or she demonstrates. If the warrior begins to view him or herself as a "choker," he or she creates a self-fulfilling prophecy that will ensure further PCA. A trainer or a leader can be extremely helpful in showing the warrior that it is only one part of performance and can be viewed as a challenge for improvement rather than a permanent scar.

6. *As your time allows, try to schedule periodic individual meetings that focus on the issue of mental training.*

Once again, don't underestimate the power of this gesture. You are letting your warriors know that you view their mental training as important and you are there to help them in that regard. Most importantly, it breaks down the barrier that warriors may feel to always present themselves as mentally tough 100% of the time. Such meetings may remove concern warriors may have about being an imposter around you, constantly fearing what will happen "if Sarge finds out what I am really like." Let them know that dedicating time to their weaknesses as well as strengths will not jeopardize their position but contribute to their potential as a warrior.

Motivation

To become elite in any high demand pursuit requires hours upon hours of training and more importantly...conditioning. Often this training and conditioning is rigorous, painful, and injurious. However, individuals who have reached the pinnacle of their pursuit have more than likely put in their time training to achieve that high level of success. To do this, these individuals must have something that motivates them to continually push their minds and their bodies, and come back from whatever struggles or setbacks they may have experienced along the way. This motivation may come intrinsically or extrinsically. Intrinsic motivation is an individual's personal drive to achieve their goal. This may be setting an organizational record, winning a competition or beating a personal best. Extrinsic motivation is the resulting motivation from an outside source such as peers, trainers, supervisors and even family.

Research has shown the link between extremely high levels of motivation and the achievement of elite status (Hardy and Parfit, 1994; Mahoney et al., 1987; Orlick and Partington, 1988). This would seem to be an obvious conclusion. There are many people out there who have the talent to succeed, even excel. In light of this, it appears that intrinsic motivation may be the greater determinant of achieving success in high performance activities. This stance is supported by several research studies (Hardy and Parfit, 1994; Mahoney et al., 1987; Orlick and Partington, 1988). To achieve an elite level in any discipline, an individual absolutely must have the motivation to train hard on a consistent basis and to overcome any obstacles or setbacks that they might face in reaching or maintaining that level of performance.

Overall, it would appear that the following traits would be common among the elite: extreme self-confidence, low performance anxiety, and high motivation. These three things are very closely related and would seem to form a cyclic pattern. For example, the individual that is highly motivated to succeed knows the importance of physical preparation and that motivation carries over to training. As a result, the individual is well-conditioned and physically prepared to meet the demands of an event. Because the warrior is physically prepared, he or she gains confidence in knowing that they have done what they need to do, and that they are physically prepared. This high confidence level carries over and results in decreased anxiety because the warrior knows that they have put in the time, are prepared, and are confident in their chances of success. Now the warrior is primed to achieve the desired results. If the warrior meets or exceeds expectations and achieves a level of success, this fuels the warrior's motivation to train and to return to or exceed that level again. Elite performers have shown a strong need to demonstrate their personal competence and self-determination As a result, they commit themselves to difficult and demanding goals. When these goals are achieved, the warrior's feelings of self-competence are conformed and their intrinsic motivation is enhanced (Hardy et al. 1996).

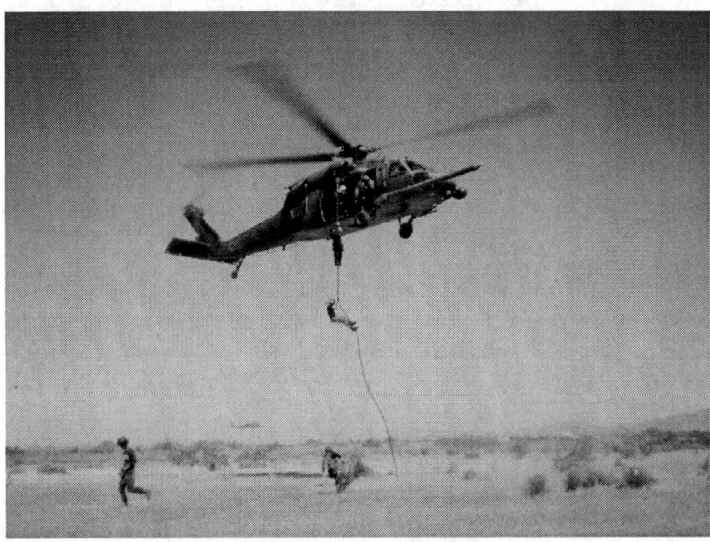

Warriors who have reached the pinnacle of their pursuit have put in the time training to achieve that high level of success. A high level of confidence that breeds success also creates a high degree of motivation to continue achieving.

Self-mastery

The warrior's ability to maintain control of mental and emotional factors is crucial for real performance, as well as establishing a psychological basis for high confidence and long-term well-being (dealing with the after-effects of a harrowing event) (Boyd & Zernong, 1999). When an individual has created a level of self-mastery or ability to control oneself, it serves to enhance all other factors of performance (Wuff & Toole, 1999). However, when warriors lose the ability to control their psychological state, especially during times of extreme stress or incapacitation, there is a serious, potentially lethal, decrease in self-confidence, well-being and even future performance (Rotella & Heyman, 1986). Because of this, productive mental skills training needs to aim at developing self-mastery. This is sired through self-knowledge that is focused at enhancing the psychological state of the warrior, in other words...Training to Win!

Like any form of training, the various methods to develop self-knowledge require time, distinct and definite goals and the willingness of the warrior to make it happen! A significant level of motivation is essential for success in the endeavor, much more than what is required for physical or mechanically-based skills, that have actual quantifiable results. Mental skills training requires a real degree of patience and trust, especially since results are not readily apparent or visible. Oftentimes, I am teaching a brief 3-day class on some sort of typical tactical skill, like tactical handgun. I will usually have the cross mix of students, some who are excited to be there at the prospect of doing something different, some who are there to have their existing skill validated and don't think they will learn anything new, and some who were ordered to be there by their agency...it could be a party at the Playboy mansion and they still wouldn't want to be there! When I start a class I'll ask, "Who here thinks that in 24 hours of training, I will have made a significant impact on you and been able to change your behavior?" Many will raise their hands and I will tell them, "Well...you're wrong! The best I can do is give you some tools that you can use to possibly change your own behavior and even with that, for me to give you the most I can, I need all of you to take this short class as seriously as you can and look at all of it with an open mind!"

Creating and sustaining individual motivation with patience and persistence is crucial from beginning to end!

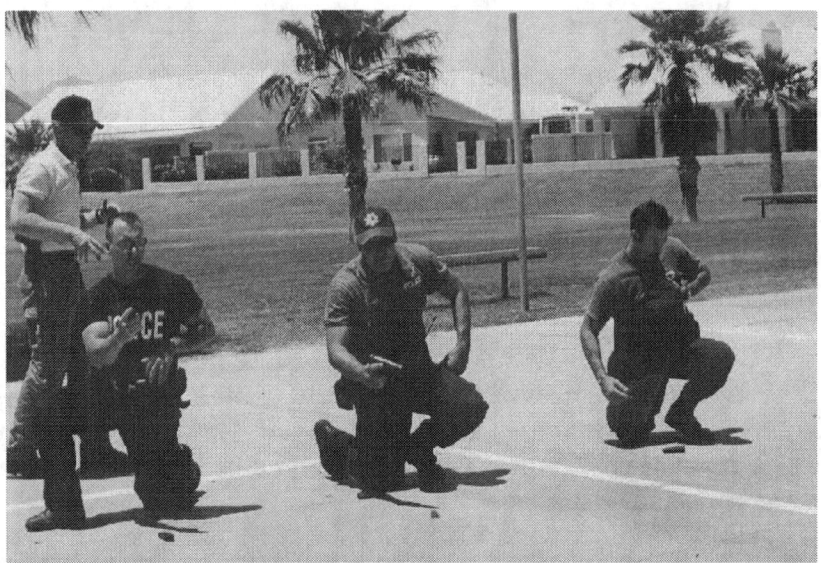

Self-mastery is sired through self-knowledge that is focused at enhancing the psychological state of the warrior, in its most basic concept...Training to Win!

Methods of Mental Skill Training

Most mental skills training techniques can be lumped into two basic categories, cognitive and somatic. Cognitive methods include mental rehearsals and visualization (imagery). Somatic methods include bio-feedback and meditation. Although cognitive and somatic methods develop the psychological side of the warrior from differing perspectives, there is considerable overlap because of the nature of the psychosomatic function. This means that components of each tend to saturate elements of the others, but it's useful to characterize each separately as it helps to explain the different aspects of human nature and performance-based psychology.

Cognitive Methods

Schema Theory

The Schema Theory, developed by Schmidt (1975, 1976), described movement as being primarily controlled by pre-programmed commands and generalized motor patterns that are pulled out of the subconscious and executed on demand. However, once these commands are executed, especially during some sort of quick movement, they require no interruption by sensory information (controlled by the subconscious). If the conscious mind interferes, then the motor pattern becomes corrupted and malformed. This is because conscious intervention is too slow to manage required alterations in coordination; this competition between the conscious and subconscious is the basis for what is generally characterized as "choking." By using mental training skills, especially imagery and visualization, the motor pattern can be practiced and more refined and a tendency of intervention by the conscious mind at critical times is reduced considerably.

Stages of Motor Learning

Similar to Schema Theory and introduced by Fitts and Posner (1964, 1967), it describes the stages of motor learning in three phases:

1. **The Cognitive Phase**, consciously learning a new skill

2. **The Associative Phase**, where minor adjustments are made to the new skill in an attempt to perfect it.

3. **The Autonomous Phase**, this is when mastery of the new skill reaches a point where it can be executed unconsciously.

In this theory, it is suggested that even if the cognitive and associative phases are properly performed, the autonomous phase may not be adequately reinforced within the mind to allow for unconscious activation. Practiced mental skills can establish the level of reinforcement to allow for the subconscious retrieval of the skill. If not, there still exists a high potential for the conscious mind to interfere, slowing down the process and destroying coordination and ability, and creating a life-threatening situation.

The Set Hypothesis

This hypothesis suggests that before a successful motor skill can be executed, a specific internal state is required, allowing for optimal coordination of activation (Nascon & Schmidt, 1971), especially after extended periods of no training, practice or use. This is consistent with the state of affairs for most law enforcement agencies where training may occur on an infrequent basis (once a month, once a quarter, once a year, etc). Adjustments in arousal and attention need to be modified depending on the particular task and this needs to be repeated each time. By rehearsing this aspect of skill performance internally, the warrior can practice bringing forth the psychological conditions needed for performance. If not, then before the skill has a chance of execution, the risk of failure grows higher because the essential psychological conditions don't occur and optimal performance is not possible.

Depending on the nature of the task (closed skill or open skill) and the skill level of the individual warrior, the advantages of mental rehearsal and other mental skills are twofold.

First, mental skills can reinforce unconscious processes responsible for executing enhanced skill efficiency (Cohn, 1990). This is because conscious control of quick and/or complicated movements are too slow, meaning it takes the conscious mind too long to come up with a solution to a problem, and thus contribute significantly to destruction of intended action and movements (choking).

Second, initiation of specific arousal and attention processes, linking of stimulus to response. Therefore, the motor skill component and the pre-skill or pre-performance build-up need to be rehearsed for efficient and appropriate response.

Lobmeyer and Wasserman (1986) investigated pre-performance training routines on elite athletes. Subjects in the investigation showed a 7% increase in performance during practice sessions when using a pre-performance routine versus those who did not. Wrisberg and Anshel (1989) found that mental imagery in conjunction with arousal control was a highly effective pre-performance strategy to enhance the performance of athletes. Moore (1986) evaluated the effects of an overt/covert routine training program on adherence to, and performance of, a pre-performance routine for athletes. Overt or behavioral based strategies such as practicing mechanical skills (swinging a stick, pulling a trigger) and covert or cognitive based strategies (mental skills) were used. The study showed that athletes adherence to a pre-performance routine increased performance and reaction time. Interviews with the athletes involved indicated a positive effect on confidence and self-esteem, as well as enhanced aggressiveness.

An additional advantage of mental skills training is the absence of major physical exertion that the individual warrior would have to perform under traditional training regimes. This can alleviate the risk of overtraining, that is a constant supply of anxiety among many individuals and agencies (Warr, 1996). Mental skills training has been demonstrated to be an effective tool to increase performance and the ability to recover. Understand that there are a great many methods and techniques in mental skills training; this book covers many of the most fundamental methods.

Chapter Two

TRAINING THE MIND AND THE BODY

"I am not one of those who think that coming in second or third is winning."

— Robert Francis Kennedy

I t really doesn't take much physical fitness or strength to be a good police officer, at least in the model sense of the modern community-oriented officer so highly sought by contemporary agencies. However, it does to be a warrior. This includes self-motivation, self-discipline and a willingness to take on new challenges. Within the realm of the warrior there are many different tasks and functions that have one thing in common, they require an extraordinary grasp of attentional, emotional and physical skills, often all applied at the same time and under some very arduous conditions.

Greater than any other calling, the life of the warrior requires mental skills in combination with physical or mechanical skills. Yet, mental training is an area which has been long neglected in the fields of conflict management and force application. A mental training program for any endeavor involves learning to apply skills that include, goal-setting, self-talk, imagery and concentration. Many recent studies have indicated conclusively that a structured mental training program can greatly improve performance. Another interesting finding is that the more a task requires pure skill rather than elements of power and endurance, the more likely it will be that mental skills played a strong role in the success of that task.

What Exactly Is Mental Training?

Mental training is the learning, practicing and application of mental and psychological skills through:

- Short term and long term goals
- Reframing negative thought patterns to positive thoughts and belief systems
- Making positive affirmations
- Relaxation
- Visualization and imagery
- Concentration and attentional focusing

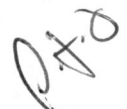

Any warrior involved in a conflict management, force application or situational control situations could benefit greatly from these skills, whether a rookie or a seasoned veteran.

The basic assumption of mental training programs is that our imagination has great power; that we create our reality through the things which we think about, whether positive or negative. The idea is to focus on the positive and eliminate the negative. It has been suggested that through use of mental training, warriors can change attitudes, motivate themselves, expedite the learning of new skills, increase levels of performance and identify problems they may be having with a specific aspect of their performance. However, it is only in recent years that we have had strong scientific evidence that supports these ideas.

We do not perform physical skills in isolation without mental skills; therefore, we have to approach our performance from more of a holistic perspective in order to integrate the mental and physical aspects of performance and achieve our fullest potential. Peak performance doesn't just happen. It occurs because many factors that contribute to producing performance all come together. The only way to determine the pattern for that performance is to record all the things leading up to it; having established a pattern of preparation, you can increase the likelihood of being able to make it happen on a regular basis.

As the awareness and recognition of mental training increases it becomes obvious that all training programs should incorporate psychological principles with the same emphasis and degree as those placed on physiological and mechanical principles. What is required for mental training to be effective is practice, development, and regular, systematic application.

Mental training teaches the warrior to interpret what is happening and why, how to cope with whatever is encountered and how to make logical and appropriate decisions based on relevant cues. Warriors need to learn these skills and strategies in order to achieve consistent performance even under the worst conditions.

Enhancing Performance

Performance enhancement is the deliberate cultivation of an effective perspective on achievement and the systematic use of a combination of effective cognitive skills and physical/mechanical skills. A warrior can maximize his or her performance by mastering habits and emotional and physical states. Most of the training methods for this cultivation are derived from applied sport psychology used in professional and elite athletes, and are highly applicable to other forms of human performance, including the development of warriors.

Using the mind's power to find an edge has become an indispensable element in training modern athletes. The transformation of warriors is similar in many respects to the changes and challenges that occur in elite athletes, but to date there has been no real body of professionals dedicated to training mental skills in warriors and war fighters—until now. The staff at The Khyber Training Group, has been committed to state of the art training of warriors of all walks (Law enforcement, Military, Security, etc) in applied psychology in combination with intense mechanical and physical training. Khyber has been committed to intense training and conditioning since 1992. Offering students a unique taste of success and performance enhancement.

Elements of Enhanced Performance

The concepts of training and conditioning to win integrate five key elements of applied psychology into a systematic approach to empower individual warriors and organizations, including:

Cognitive Foundations

Understanding the psychology of high performance (the zone) and knowing how the mind works, allowing the warrior to gain confidence and operate in the most efficient manner. Skills include: positive self-talk, restructuring ineffective beliefs, and cultivating a powerful self-image.

Goal Setting

Goal setting (chapter three) is the process of identifying the underlying rationale for performance, then creating action plans for attaining goals.

Attention Control

Attention control (chapter seven) includes selectively attending to important cues, shifting the field of awareness and developing simple procedures and routines that streamline the execution of repetitive tasks to attain optimum focus and concentration.

Stress Management

Understanding how stress operates in the human system (chapter nine) and mastering techniques of recovery and energy management as a preemptive antidote for burnout and fatigue.

Imagery and Visualization

The process of seeing, feeling and experiencing desired outcomes and taking actions to attain them (chapter four), building confidence (chapter six) and team and individual readiness to carry on.

These competencies improve individual and team performance by empowering individuals to:

- Create effective thinking habits and perform with realistic confidence
- Improve attentional skills
- Control physical, emotional, and mental responses to high-stress, high-performance demands
- Operate with a sense of clarity regarding immediate actions and mitigating long-term situations.

When warriors train in a full performance enhancement environment their training maximizes their performance for involvement in real-world events. Further, they condition to improve physical skills, confidence, and control skills.

Improving the Edge

True warriors are hungry for knowledge and skills to improve their edge in real-world events, so much to the point that we have dozens of warrior-based training competitions held all over the world, competitions pitting team against team and man against man, all symbolizing a test of the warriors' abilities.

The balance of mind, body, spirit and emotions may sound metaphysical or spiritual in nature. However, it is, in all reality, the foundation for the mental skills and associated training philosophy for truly conditioning warriors to win.

The following chapters in this book describe a program that enables the warrior to achieve peak performance by using mental training tools and skills. Instructions for using these tools, along with several different examples, are interwoven throughout the book. Each chapter will provide information that helps a warrior develop skills to use the various mental tools.

Mental training skills may sound and appear simple, but they are extremely powerful. When a warrior sets goals, what he says to himself and what he sees, and doesn't see, are vitally important to the warrior's success and long-term stability.

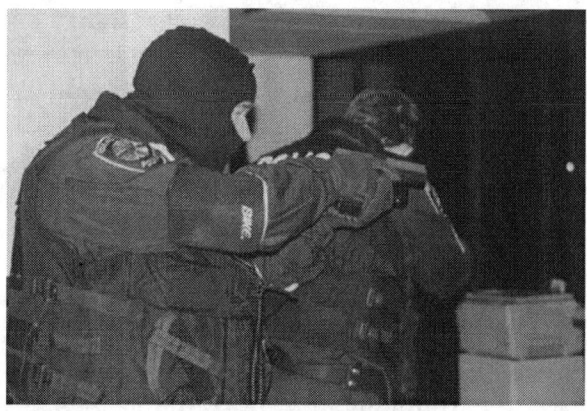

True warriors are hungry for knowledge, skills, and experiences to improve their edge.

Why Would Warriors Not Use Mental Training?

If so many warriors can be helped by the support provided through solid psychological training and are aware of its benefits, why don't more of them seek out this type of training? In a word, why do they resist the benefits of this type of training and how can we change this situation?

Resistance is a concept with a long history in psychoanalysis, yet literally no history in performance-based psychology. The field of performance or applied sports psychology has been dominated by the concepts of cognitive behaviorism and in reality resistance to training is a phenomenon they have paid very little attention to. What has happened over time is a circumvention of sorts when faced with resistance, where an emphasis has been placed on the length of training, resulting in shorter training sessions as a means of dealing with resistance. Resistance has been characterized as the culmination of the various forces within an individual that create opposition to anything new (Greenson, 1967). Despite suffering all the maladies associated with performance, like: inhibition, anxiety, depression and even alcoholism, warriors will only turn to psychology as a last resort. Studies throughout the country suggest that at least 10%-15% of the population suffer from these various conditions at any given time and these folks don't have the outside stressors that professional warriors do.

Most folks that fall within the Warrior class, who have these problems, refuse to deal with them and literally suffer in silence. Freud suggested that resistance to any treatment stemmed from guilt, the need to suffer, secondary gains brought on by the symptoms, habit and repetitive compulsions (Freud, 1926). Freud's concepts were established with the average man in mind, not taking into consideration the specific issues and dynamics associated with warriors. When shifting this concept to the performance psychology field, we need to take into consideration all of the various dynamics of warriors and one in particular, narcissism (Kohut, 1977). Narcissism is an affliction common to the various warrior classes in our society, characterized with colorful terms like: Alpha male, Alpha female, John Wayne, Jane Wayne, etc. Narcissists have been found to be especially resistant to many things considered "out of the box," because of an innate unwillingness to become dependent on others. Warriors, be they cops or soldiers, have been shown to be aloof, aggressive, driven and very independent, fitting the textbook description of the narcissist to a T (Russell, 1993).

Ways of Resisting

The following is a brief explanation of the most common methods warriors use to resist. Given the very common experience of anxiety and anger that warriors feel and how they manage it on their own, I suggest that warriors use the following four methods to manage their uncontrolled affect.

1. Superstitious Behavior

It is very common to see or hear warriors using some sort of ritualistic behavior. From the warrior's perspective, these superstitions are necessary for performance and good luck. The ritual can be beneficial as a part of pre-event preparation routine, distracting the warrior from mounting anxiety and provides a sense of control. These various rituals are often accepted by teammates, trainers, and administrators. They are common. I, myself, wear a good luck charm made from an amulet given to me by a martial arts master I trained with in Korea and one of my oldest daughter's baby rings. This charm is around my neck every day. Further, I wear a braided bracelet that belonged to a close friend, that was given to me by his mother the day his body was brought home from Afghanistan.

2. Performance enhancement and stress control through drugs

A dramatically more dangerous way to control perform- ance is through the use of chemicals. This growing epidemic in all performance-oriented pursuits is another example of individuals avoiding training and support instead of attempt- ing to manage emotions in a self-defeating manner. The warrior who suffers from anxiety, depression, pain or fatigue will often turn to chemicals for help, even if it's illegal and dangerous (Wadler & Hainline, 1989).

3. Eating and drinking disorders

Many warriors, particularly those working where physical fitness and weight standards must be maintained, will starve themselves to achieve what is perceived as the ideal weight (Bailey, 1998). The uneducated warrior will actually ignore food to get in shape.

4. Exercise bulimia

Another way warriors try to manage anxiety, anger, shame, or poor self-image is through over-training. The sad part of this problem is that they will often combine this method with chemical use, eating disorders, or alcoholism which can actually worsen the conditions considerably.

A twenty-man section of elite athletes was approached by a team of research psychologists. Each subject was asked to fill out an eleven item questionnaire which took about 10 minutes to complete. The group consisted of 17 males and 3 females. There were 6 golf professionals, 6 long distance runners, 4 Olympic swimmers, 1 tennis pro, 1 professional basketball player, 1 fitness trainer, and 1 professional football player. The questionnaire contained questions that asked about their familiarity with performance psychology, if they had ever embraced the benefits of performance psychology, if they felt they could benefit from performance psychology and why they had not used performance psychology. The questionnaire provided the following results:

- Two had been in training with a performance psychology specialist
- Two conceded that their sports pursuits were 50% mental
- Eighteen felt there was a negative stigma involved in working with performance psychology
- Sixteen felt they could personally benefit considerably from performance psychology
- All twenty agreed that performance psychology was an important and neglected facet of training.

Only 10% of those polled admitted to having trained with performance psychology which is roughly the same number as the section of society with emotional problems in the U.S., yet 100% agreed that performance psychology was important to training. This poll supports the suggestion that warriors and the athletically elite will resist the mental side of training. Those polled thought nothing of investing personal time and money in equipment they felt would enhance their performance, but were unwilling to consider mental performance enhancement. In the United States, warriors from all walks invest roughly $3000+ per year in training that they perceive as important and enjoyable. So on the surface the information doesn't make a lot of sense. They invest heavily in the profession and in the needs they feel are important, they understand that a tremendous amount of their job is psychological and that they could benefit from mental skills training, yet only a small percentage actually take advantage of it. The resistance to this type of training is not entirely conscious. Most of those polled were never queried about their emotions. Sure they were asked and freely talked about mental training, focus, concentration, visualization, and perform-ance enhancement, but there was never mention of how they felt. It's really difficult to understand how individuals with obvious needs for performance growth and enhancement have inhibitions to that function, admitting that it is of great benefit to them, but failing to utilize it.

Just by taking part in a simple in-service training session, it is clear that individuals, especially the macho, narcissistic folks in our realm, get defensive against the use of specialized training sessions, just as much as they do over seeing a counselor when they have experienced something bad. Possibly from fear of failure or fear of embarrassment. After all, the performance in our occupations is all about action and the discharge of emotion through movement rather than through words. Sitting in a chair or lying on a couch, being immobile, allowing things to come up from the subconscious can be terrifying (though no one will admit it). We can talk all we want about performance enhancement and performance psychology, but without applying it in a working environment it is a hard sell. Applying the skills mentioned in this book are done easily in an active, training environment. As training specialists, this is our playing field, it is our job and our function to bridge this gap, to bring the mental side of training to the active training environment and to integrate these trains of thought. Just understand, that as you try to implement this type of training, you may find that they fear you much more than an armed crack-head on the street. If we manage to break down that fear, we will create an environment that will provide the warrior with much more than ever before and create a tool that they will actually apply.

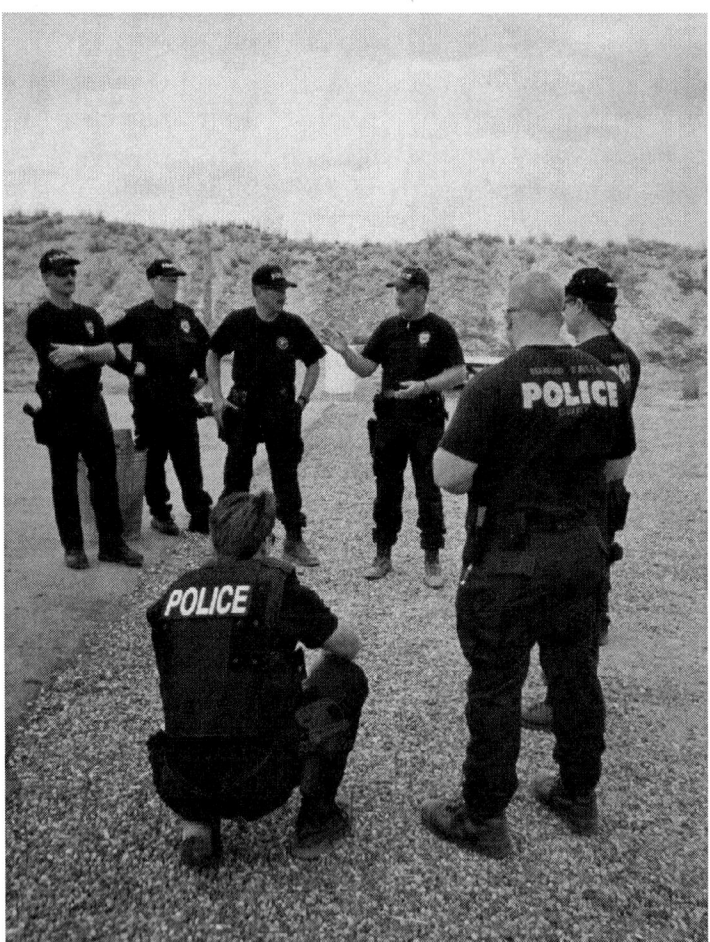

Warriors can and frequently will, resist concepts like mental training. This occurs for a number of reasons, it is a major challenge that trainers must overcome.

Chapter Three

GOAL SETTING: DETERMINE WHERE YOU WANT TO GO

"To solve a problem or to reach a goal, you don't need to know all the answers in advance. But you must have a clear idea of the problem or the goal you want to reach."
— W. Clement Stone

Let's Take a Journey

Goal setting is a process that **CAN** help in the pursuit of a destination, any destination, especially the pursuit of training and performance excellence. Goal setting is the basis of all mental conditioning programs and quality goal setting should always be part of the warrior's mental conditioning plan. Goal setting provides a structure for motivation and direction. Basically you must know where you want to go if you are to have a reasonable chance of getting there.

Goals are not something we make judgments about, they are simply things which we choose to pursue and achieve. Whatever the warriors' goals, they must be specific to the individual or to the organization; things that individuals strive to attain for their own or group satisfaction, rather than because someone else attained them sooner.

Starting the Journey

Before we start or can get anywhere, a little planning needs to be done. Where exactly are we going? Let's plot a cross-country course through Southern Utah, like running a high performance expedition race! How are we going to get from the starting line to the finish? How will we get from check point to check point? What routes are we going to take? What supplies are we going to need for the race? Food, equipment repair material, medical supplies, of course (this is based on first-hand experience, trust me), quality footwear, safety equipment....

But, let's not forget the map. The easiest way to plan for any excursion is with a good map. When using a map you are in essence setting goals for the expedition.

The road map can:

- locate specifically where it is you are going (long-term goal)
- determine how many planned stops to take along the way (short-term goal)
- tell you how many miles to the next destination (daily goal)
- tell you the alternate routes along the way

Now, let's apply this to the realm of training, specifically as it pertains to the demanding world of use of force and force application skills. Similar questions should be asked of warriors before they take off on an intense training pursuit. Where will they want to be at the end of the evolution? What are they going to do physically and mentally in order to get there? What skills and tools do they need in order to reach their destination? This application of mental skills, done in conjunction with physical and mechanical skills, will help warriors plan their training and conditioning journey with consistent use of goals. The chapter contains a brief introduction, tips on the presentation of goal setting to individuals and teams and some exercises to help build the training and conditioning road map.

How Exactly Does Goal Setting Help?

Good goal setting gives an athlete an edge in three areas.

> **Goals...**
>
> Provide direction
> Provide feedback
> Motivate; provide a daily purpose

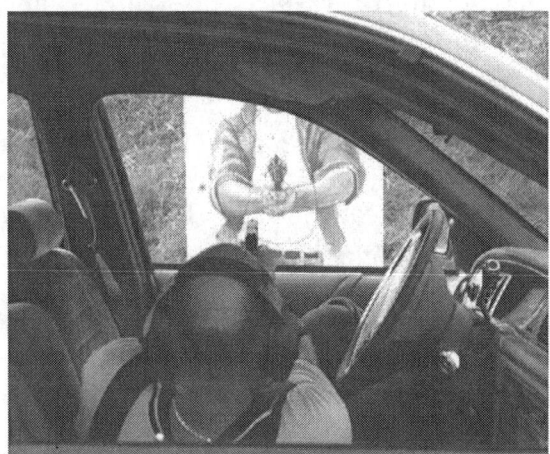

Goal setting is the basis of all mental
conditioning programs and quality goal
setting should always be part of the warrior's
mental conditioning plan.

Basics of Effective Goal Setting

1. Identify Both Short- and Long-term Goals

When planning a mission, you often think about specific
details. Where do you go to obtain certain resources? Who has
what abilities? Determining these constitutes parts of very short-
term goals.

Warriors need to progress from short-term goals to long-term
goals. Long-term goals are typically quarterly or annual goals,
possibly even a few years. One way to determine a good long-
term goal would be to have your warriors ask themselves the
question, "Where do I want to be at the end of the year or the end
of the quarter?" Examples of the answer to this question can be
in terms of having an improved performance, better qualifications scores, beating a specific standard, or making selection to
a spot on a team.

In order to make the long-term goal seem less intimidating,
short-term goals are set. Short-term goals are set for shorter
lengths of time than long-term goals, usually between a week and
a month. Short-term goals serve as stepping stones for the long-

term goals. Setting short-term goals allow one to monitor success towards the long-term goals. The question here is, "Where do I want to be at the end of this period?"

Lastly, short-term goals can also often feel far off, therefore, something more within reach is needed to maintain focus and motivation. For these reasons it is also important to set daily goals. Daily goals are to be set every day in training and in operational events. Setting effective daily goals will help motivate and bring higher intensity to training. Daily goals can be set for both physical and psychological skill development. The question here is, "Why am I doing what I am doing today?"

2. Identify Task Goals in Addition to Outcome Goals

Most individuals are good at setting outcome goals; an outcome goal is any type of goal directed at the end result. Warrior-based outcome goals are set when an individual focuses on attaining a specific end result, arresting the suspect, saving the hostage, or making the arrest. Outcome goals are hard to control because they depend on both the ability and skill of the warrior and his opponents.

However, the individual has the most control over task goals because they depend on their own skills and abilities only. Task goals are what the warrior has to do (physically and mentally) in order to accomplish outcome goals. Examples of task goals include being aggressive on corners and barricades, maintaining a specific speed on approach or temp throughout an exercise.

3. Take Action

For the most part, with little or no support, warriors are already setting goals. When asked, most individuals will talk about goals such as wanting to score higher on a specific assessment, higher qualification scores and higher PT scores. However, trainers and leaders need to help warriors progress from setting goals to actually acting on their goals.

For example, when John, a 10-year veteran of his agency's tactical unit, starts his shift he wonders if any of his goals are consequential. Does he focus on specifics in training? Or is he "just training," merely there doing what the trainers ask him to do, doing just enough to get by.

Once a goal setting "map" is established, the next crucial piece is to keep the warrior accountable to those goals. Doing this is primarily a matter of creativity and finding a means of accountability that will function for your warriors.

Examples of methods to keep goals at the vanguard, so they are acted upon, include:

- Complete regular goal setting forms

- Develop a goal tracking chart

- Write goals on visible items

- Verbalize goals to teammates, co-workers, family

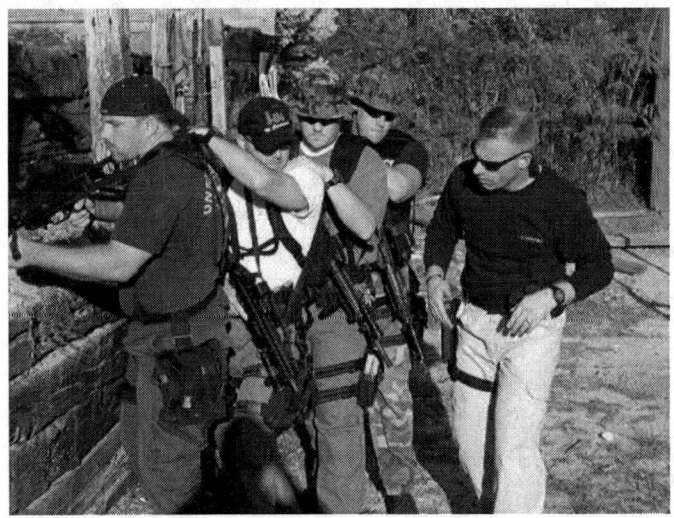

Most warriors are already setting goals, usually with little guidance. However, trainers and leaders need to help warriors progress from setting goals to actually acting on their goals.

4. Evaluate Your Goals

Once a warrior has decided what his or her goals are, continue the process by reviewing and updating. Goals are there to give direction, feedback on progress and to motivate. To ensure that goals serve these purposes, goals must also be flexible. This is why evaluation and modification is so important. Set specific dates or time periods for your warriors to monitor success and to amend goals if needed.

5. Set Both Organization and Individual Goals

The goal setting terms thus far have all been in reference to individual goals. Individual goals are very important, but in law enforcement, military or security fields we generally operate in a team format. It is extremely important to set goals for the team. Team goals define a desirable state for a group at the end of a specific period of time. Team goals can guide how individual goals are set. Both warriors and trainers can be included in the team goal setting process. If the trainer sets the overall team goals, it is important to include the warriors in setting the group goals for their specific team function or sub-team. After the group goals are set, the warriors can then set their individual goals as a reflection of the group and team goals.

TRAINER'S GUIDE

- Ask your warriors to define goals. Have them discuss why they set goals. Then, discuss additional ways that goals can help performance.
- Teach your warriors the importance of systematic goal setting (using different lengths and types of goals) and give examples of other warriors to stress the point.
- Discuss, in detail, the tips of effective goal setting as outlined in this chapter.
- Have your warriors complete some of the goal setting exercises at the end of this chapter.
- Brainstorm ways for the team to "Stay on top of" the goal setting plan.

Goal Setting Exercises

To help your warriors understand and use goals more often, in training and in the real world, several goal setting worksheets and recording sheets have been included. Feel free to pick and choose which ones work best for you and your individual situation. The sheets have been included to get warriors started on effective goal setting; feel free to modify the forms by incorporating your own ideas into your goal setting program.

- **Exercise 1 and 2**

  These are targeted at older more seasoned warriors; they are designed to bring home the differences between short- and long-term goals and outcome and task goals.

- **Exercise 3**

  This is an example of a goal setting sheet for operational events and can be used with any experience level. Write the name of the event in the first blank given. Choose a goal time for each event, remembering to keep them challenging and realistic. Keep the sheet in a safe place and remember to review it before a real world operation (time and circumstances permitting).

- **Exercise 4, 5, and 6**

  These exercises are targeted towards newer, less experienced warriors. The main purpose of these exercises is to get the newer warriors thinking about short- and long-term goals and emphasize how one type of goal influences others.

- **Exercise 7**

  This exercise can be used with any experience level. Setting and recording daily goals is important. Daily goals can be recorded in many different ways; one method is recording daily goals on 3x5 cards.

- **Exercise 8**

This exercise is designed for creating individual's goals as a reflection of team goals. Once your warriors have set group goals for a specific time period, have them set goals for further progress towards group and team goals. Then ask your warriors what they can do daily as individuals to further progress towards the group and team goals.

Finally, at the end of this chapter, some training log templates have been included in more detail.

GOAL SETTING - Exercise 1
How far should I look ahead?

Long-term goals tell you where you want to go and short-term goals tell you how your going to get there. Both are equally important for effective goal setting. Try this exercise to help you breakdown your long-term goals.

1. *What is one of your long-term goals for the set time period?*

2. *What are the abilities or skills you will need to achieve this goal?*

    a.
    b.
    c.

3. *What can you do between now and the end of the time period to develop abilities and skills?*

    a.
    b.
    c.

4. *What will you do this week to develop those abilities and skills?*

    a.
    b.
    c.

5. *What can you do during your next training cycle to develop those abilities and skills?*

    a.
    b.
    c.

GOAL SETTING - Exercise 2
Moving beyond outcome goals to task goal setting

Outcome goals tell you where you want to be, which can help motivate. But, on a daily basis, they do not tell you what you need to do.

1. Start with an outcome

Choose an upcoming event (training or planned operation) and pick a challenging but not impossible outcome goal. Write that goal down in detail here:

2. Moving from outcome to task goals

How can you maximize your chances to achieve this goal? Write down three things you can do during the event in order to increase your odds of achieving the outcome goal.

a. I will: _____

b. I will: _____

c. I will: _____

3. Practicing the task goals in training

What can you do in training between now and your listed event to increase your chances of achieving your three tasks? Write down two things to focus on in training that will gear you towards your task goals.

a. I will: _____

b. I will: _____

GOAL SETTING - Exercise 3
Setting goals for real world events

Name:

Date of event:

Name or designator of event:

Event:

Goal:

Skills needed to achieve goal:

What am I going to work on in training to help me achieve
this goal:

Name:

Date of event:

Name or designator of event:

Event:

Goal:

Skills needed to achieve goal:

What am I going to work on in training to help achieve
this goal:

GOAL SETTING - Exercise 4
Stepping stones

Write your long-term goal in the oval. The arrows all point towards the goal. Use the arrows as stepping stones and write down your short-term goals that will lead to your long-term goal.

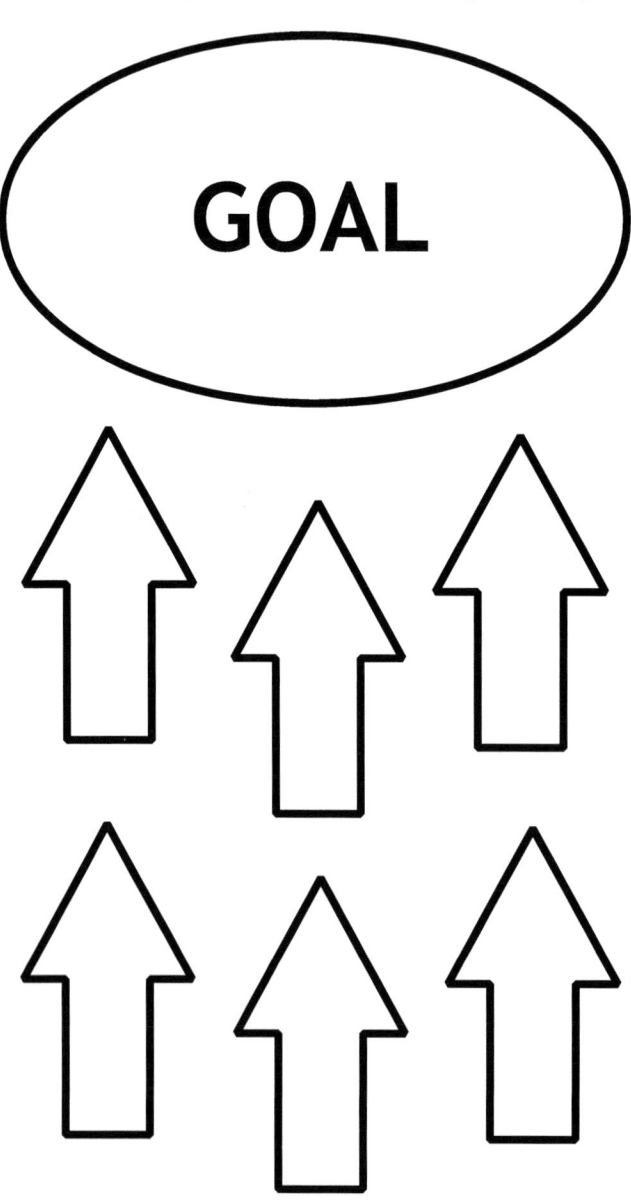

GOAL SETTING - Exercise 5
Turn goals into reality

In the box provided, write down your goals as a warrior. Then underneath it write down four things you can do today in training to bring you closer to obtaining those goals.

GOAL LIST

FOUR THINGS I CAN DO TODAY TO HELP ACHIEVE MY GOALS:

1.

2.

3.

4.

GOAL SETTING - Exercise 6
Rising
Use the chart below to help define your goals, long-term, short-term and daily goals.

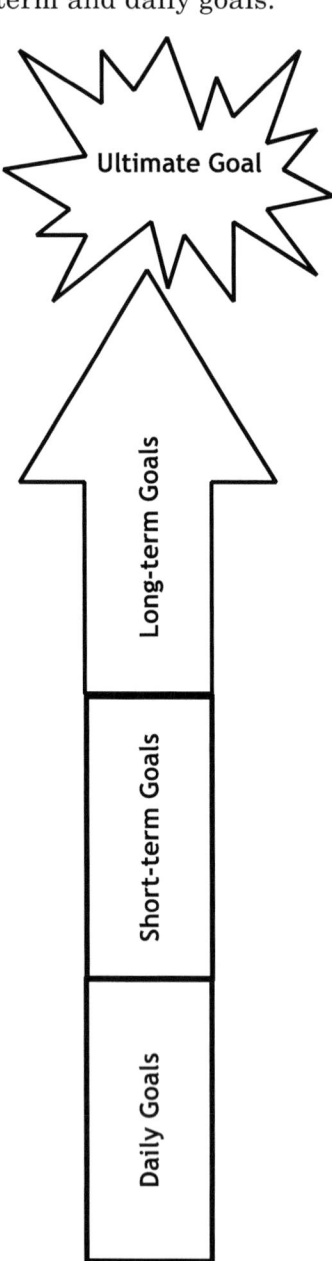

Ultimate Goals
1.
2.
Long-term Goals
Short-term Goals
1.
2.
3.
Daily Goals

GOAL SETTING - Exercise 7
Daily goal setting cards/sheet

MY GOAL FOR TODAY:

WHAT DO I NEED TO DO PHYSICALLY TO ACHIEVE MY GOAL?

1.

2.

WHAT DO I NEED TO DO MENTALLY TO ACHIEVE MY GOAL?

1.

2.

GOAL SETTING - Exercise 8
Team, Group & Individual goals

NAME:

DATE:

GROUP / TEAM:

TEAM GOAL(S) FOR: _____

1.

2.

3.

GROUP GOAL(S) FOR: _____ (WHAT CAN WE DO AS A
GROUP TO WORK TOWARDS THE TEAM GOAL(S)?)

1.

2..

3.

INDIVIDUAL GOAL(S) FOR: _____ (WHAT CAN I DO AS AN
INDIVIDUAL TO WORK TOWARDS BOTH TEAM AND GROUP
GOAL(S)?)

1.

2.

3.

Keeping Track of Progress, Training Logs

An important aspect of setting goals is writing them down and making them real. One way to help track goals is by maintaining a training log. This written log of daily or regular activities serves as a way to help maintain a more systematic focus on all aspects of training and real world events. Training logs can include information about both physical and mental practice and goals. Benefits from keeping a training log, include developing a better sense of how you spend your training time, knowing where improvements are coming from, increasing your motivation to keep working hard, and heightening your awareness during real-world operational events.

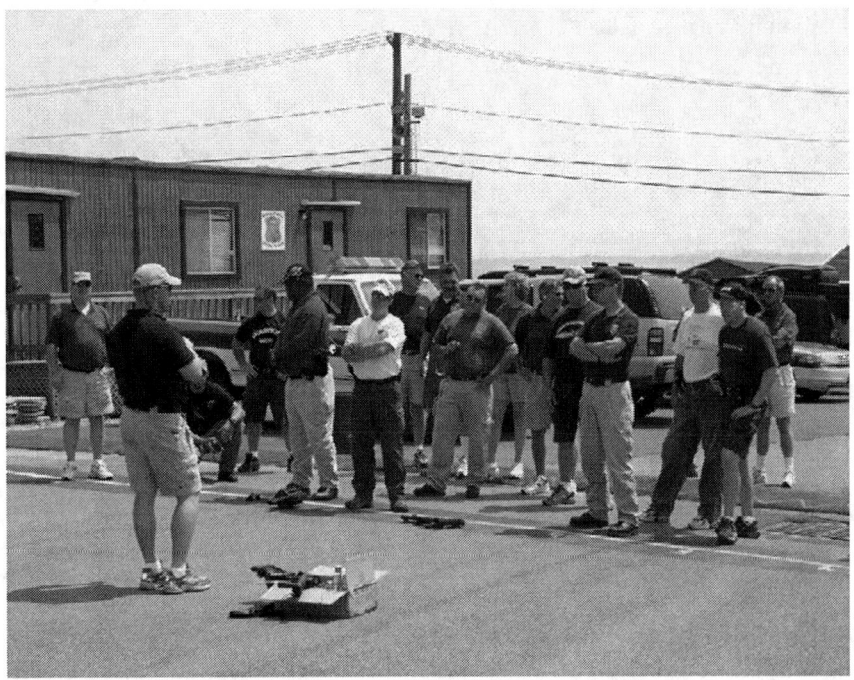

Training logs need to include information about both physical and mental practice and goals, helping warriors turn goals into realities.

Pre-training:

Physical Training Goals:

1.

2.

3.

Mental Training Goals:

1.

2.

3.

Post Training Evaluation:

Physical Training Goals - Accomplishments

Physical Training Goals - Problems

Mental Training Goals - Accomplishments

Mental Training Goals - Problems

TRAINING LOG BOOK Page 2

Date: _____

This period's goal(s):

1.

2.

3.

4.

Strategies for achieving goal(s):

1.

2.

3.

4.

Obstacles that might prevent achievement of goal(s):

1.

2.

3.

4.

Self-Evaluation:

TRAINING LOG BOOK   Page 3

Date/Time: _____

Type of training (specify):

Mental Training Goals:

Training plan/Training accomplished:

Comments:

OPERATIONAL LOG BOOK

DATE: _____

OPERATIONAL EVENT:

DATE & TIME OF EVENT:

HOW DID YOU FEEL?

TRAINER'S OR LEADER'S COMMENTS:

DATE: _____

OPERATIONAL EVENT:

DATE & TIME OF EVENT:

HOW DID YOU FEEL?

TRAINER'S OR LEADER'S COMMENTS:

Chapter Four

IMAGERY: SEE IT, BELIEVE IT AND MAKE IT HAPPEN

"Deep into that darkness peering, long I stood there, wondering, fearing, doubting, dreaming dreams no mortal ever dared to dream before."

— Edgar Allan Poe

What Exactly Is Imagery?

> **Warriors:** Take a minute and think back to your best day this year. Picture the setting where the envisioned situation took place, see your opponent, try to experience how you felt standing in the stack or on scene, recall what you were thinking the last few seconds before the call was initiated, feel your reaction as you entered into the unknown.
>
> As you thought about your best success, were you able to make the experience "real"? You may not know it, but when re-creating your past success you were using imagery, a critical skill in conditioning to win.

Mental imagery is a skill warriors can tap into to help achieve goals. It is a skill that is essential for positive conditioning. In nearly all aspects of training, as it relates to our warrior class, an individual can practice realistic rehearsals for hours. Sometimes mental imagery is referred to as visualization or mental rehearsal and it is defined as an experience that resembles a perceptual experience, but occurs in the absence of actual stimuli. Whenever we imagine ourselves performing an action in the absence of actual physical practice, we are using imagery.

Learning to conduct imagery or visualization is a skill like any other. It takes time, patience and practice. When in transit to a mission site, visualize the operation you're about to conduct. Is the image clear, detailed and accurate? For most people the answer is "Sort of," "A little," and "Kind of." Learning to use imagery will take more time than the time it takes to drive a van from a ready room to a warrant site.

Most warriors use some sort of mental imagery naturally, though often not in a purposeful way. Similar to physical and mechanical skills, mental skills like imagery need to be cultivated in various locations and under various conditions. This way the warrior can call on these skills when needed and when under pressure or stress. Many activities, in sports and in conflict management, not only rely on physical skills, but on a strong "mental" game as well. Most trainers and coaches routinely preach the buzz phrase, "It's 90% mental and 10% physical," especially in activities where success is measured in hundredths or tenths of a second, like in a fist fight or a gun fight. Because of this, a countless number of people are turning to mental imagery to take their skill performance to a higher level.

The Basis for Imagery and Visualization

The parts of the brain responsible for motor skill execution (prefrontal cortex and basal ganglia) are also responsible for the imagery process under conscious thought without actual movement being involved (Decety, 1996; Jeannerod, 1995). That is, those neural operations in- 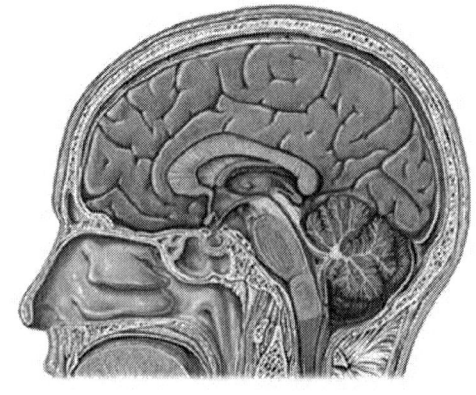 volved in motor skill execution and coordination also play a role in mentally representing those actions in conscious thought, through imagery, without generating actual movement. However, imagining an event happening is not enough to elicit the actual imagery or visualization process, and like motor skills, if the mental imagery technique is performed wrong or flawed, without sufficient attention to details, the process will be ineffective.

There are a lot of requirements in accomplishing the desired effect of imagery; the first is the approach to teaching and learning specific techniques. The visuo-spatial and temporal parts form the technical knowledge required for effective mental imagery, while conceptual (ideas) and symbolical (language) elements form the declarative knowledge of mental imagery (Annett, 1995, 1996). Technical knowledge is the knowledge of knowing how to do something, in imagery it's based on being able to form the correct image in the mind. Declarative knowledge is different because knowledge of "knowing that," or the concept or idea behind the imagery method in order to gain an understanding of the mental imagery process, and intervening conceptually, or symbolically to assist understanding. This sort of distinction has a similar foundation in "implicit" and "explicit" knowledge in cognitive psychology, in that these terms signify whether an individual knows what they are doing (explicit), compared to the individual knowing how they are doing it (implicit) (Anderson, 1980). These two forms of knowledge are critical if the warrior is to learn the techniques needed to perform mental imagery for the greatest effect. This is because imagining the skill, and actually performing the skill, need to be as closely executed as possible for effectiveness (Currie & Ravenscroft, 1997). This means that imagery requires a certain level of attention and effort to obtain the right effects.

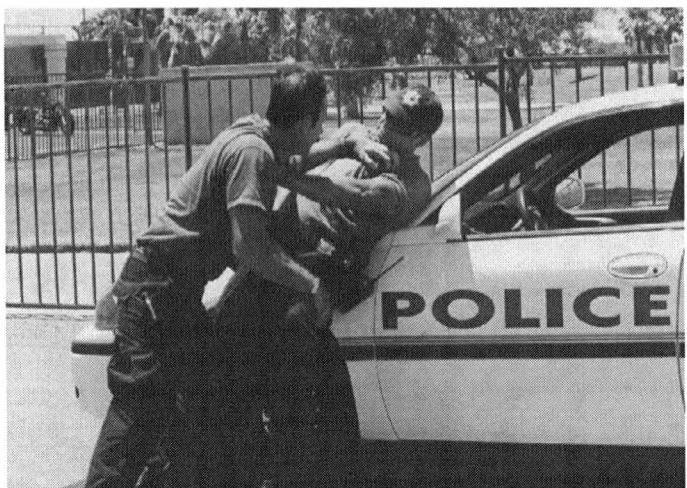

Warrior's practice imagery with the purpose of engaging as much sensory information of the actual skill as possible. That is, not only are visual and temporal senses used, but rather all the senses.

The warrior practices imagery with the goal of recruiting as much sensory information of the actual skill as possible. That is, not only are visual and temporal senses used, but rather all the senses (hearing, smell, taste and touch or body awareness). By drawing in as many senses as the warrior can that are used to perform the skill, the more realistic the simulation of imagery that can be created.

How to Implement Mental Imagery

There is no real right or wrong way to practice mental imagery. It is truly an individual pursuit. It can be done in training and in the real world, it can be short or long in duration, done sitting up, laying down, in complete silence, with music playing, eyes closed or open.

Why Imagery Works

The reason imagery works lies in the fact that when you imagine yourself perform to perfection and doing precisely what you want, you are in turn physiologically creating neural patterns in your brain, just as if you had physically performed the action. These patterns are similar to small roads embedded in the brain which can ultimately enable a warrior to perform feats by simply practicing the move mentally. Mental imagery is intended to train the brain and create the neural patterns in our brain to teach our muscles to do exactly what we want to do.

Psychologists have tried to understand the exact mechanism that cause mental imagery to work. Countless theories exist, but performance-based psychology lacks a single theory which completely explains why imagery is so effective. The earliest theory was proposed by Carpenter in 1894 and was called the psycho-neuromuscular theory. It maintains that imagery rehearsal duplicates actual motor patterns.

Another view is the symbolic learning theory. This differs from the previous that instead of imagery working due to muscle activation, imagery works from the opportunity to practice symbolic elements of a motor task, assuming that the learning obtained from imagery relates to cognitive learning. Another popular theory is Suinn's visual motor behavior rehearsal (VMBR) model which suggests that imagery should be a holistic process that includes a complete reintegration of experience. This includes visual, auditory, tactile, emotional, and kinesthetic cues. Demonstrating that physiological responses can result from a warrior's use of imagery. Suinn's method is one of the few which has good evidence to support the theory.

A more recent model, one which also places importance on psycho-physiology, goes even further by including a specific meaning for an image. This model is known as Ahsen's triple code model of imagery (ISM). According to Ahsen, there are three fundamental parts of an image. The first is that the image itself must be a centrally arousing sensation so it is more like the real world. It has all the attributes of a sensation, the only difference is it is internal. This image provides the imager with so much realism that it can enable the warrior to interact with the image as if it were real. Secondly, there exists a somatic response. Therefore, the very act of imaging results in psycho-physiological changes in the body. Finally, the third part of the image is the actual meaning of the image. Every image has a significant meaning and that specific meaning can imply something different to each individual. Since every person has a unique background and cultural framing, the actual internal image can be quite different for each individual.

How the warrior mentally rehearses or uses imagery should vary as a function of his or her skill level. A warrior who is learning a new skill, or making a technical change in an existing performance sequence or skill set will probably shift the perspective he takes back and forth between watching others performing the skill the correct way, and then mentally becoming the performer and executing the skill himself. The learner will also slow down the speed in which he performs to give himself time to make sure he is doing everything correctly. The learner should break the transition points. Initially, the transition points are the boundaries for each segment and the segments are practiced in isolation. In other words, practice specific portions of the skills at various rates and speeds.

Then as skill builds, the warrior pays more attention to ensuring that the movement between each transition point is smooth. Because the ultimate goal is to automate performance, engaging in kinesthetic rehearsal, or actually using the muscle groups while rehearsing. It's a good idea that warriors, once they become comfortable and proficient at imagery, be as active and physical as the situation and training environment will allow. The goal for a warrior is to reach the point where he or she is kinesthetically rehearsing an entire event sequence, in real time.

How Can Imagery Improve Performance?

There are a number of specific ways that this most versatile skill can help improve the performance of warriors.

To See Success

Warriors can see and feel themselves achieving goals. Helping to build confidence in the fact that these goals can be achieved.

To Motivate

It is often difficult to maintain tempo and intensity during extended training periods and both training and operational environments can be mentally taxing, to say the very least. Thoughts and images of past and future events can be very helpful in maintaining tempo and intensity.

To Manage Energy Levels

Imagery can be used to change or alter energy levels, using calming images to relax or energizing images to get psyched.

To Learn or Perfect Skills

Imagery can be a useful additional form of practice to help master particular skills and to help establish confidence in those skills. Imagery can also be used to correct errors in techniques—either by reducing complex movements to simple skills or slowing the movements down to better analyze them.

To Refocus

During training and real world situations, many distractions can occur that can prevent a warrior from maintaining optimal focus. Imagery of what to focus on can often help get an individual back on track, by reminding the warrior of what is important.

To Prepare for Real World Events

Just as a warrior needs to prepare physically for potential real world events, he needs to get mentally ready as well. The warrior can imagine being in an operational event and mentally rehearse key elements of his performance and how that performance may need to coordinate with others on a team. The warrior can also prepare for the unexpected by imaging being in a difficult situation and then see himself successfully dealing with it.

To Evaluate Performance

After a training event or an operational event, the warrior can replay the event in his head, to reinforce what was done right and to evaluate what can be improved.

To Help with Injury Recovery

Regardless of under what circumstances they occur, injuries are no fun and can result in long term mental and physical problems. However, through the use of imagery skills, warriors can help themselves in the recovery process. A warrior can use imagery to visualize healing from the specific injury; and visualize performing specific skills in their occupation to stay fresh and current.

Tips to Best Learn and Use Imagery

Be Calm and Relaxed

Imagery is most often effective when the mind is calm and the body is relaxed. If your body is tense, take some time to relax and get focused. If you get distracted while practicing imagery, let the distracting thoughts and images pass.

An Internal or External Perspective Can Be Used

An internal perspective suggests that the warrior views his image as he would from his own eyes. An external perspective of imagery is similar to watching yourself on TV or through a spectator's eye. The warrior creates and views an image as if watching a recording of himself. One perspective is really no better than the other; both internal and external are important and useful when practicing imagery skills.

Use as Many Senses as You Can

Often, warriors only use their visual sense when imaging, seeing themselves in action, but equally important is touch, sound, smell, hearing, as these are all part of a real world experience. Paying attention to detail of various senses related to the real world can provide for more realistic imagery.

Control Your Images

In addition to vividness, one must be able to control images – making certain you see and feel yourself perform as you want to perform.

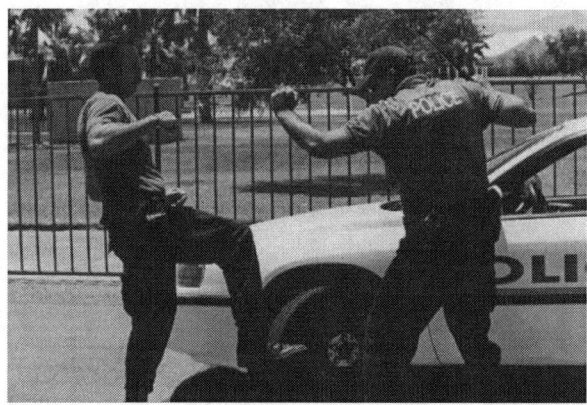

In imagery, you must see and feel yourself perform as you want to perform, controlling the image, creating the desired outcome.

Keep Imagery Simple

Start by imaging basic objects or places. Try to manipulate the image – move things. The key is to first learn how to create and re-create mental images.

Use Movement

Make images more dramatic by including movement with the imagery, this can create a full body experience to match what is being imagined—which will ultimately strengthen the image. Given the physical nature of conflict, including movements can be very helpful in increasing imagery effectiveness and overall self-awareness.

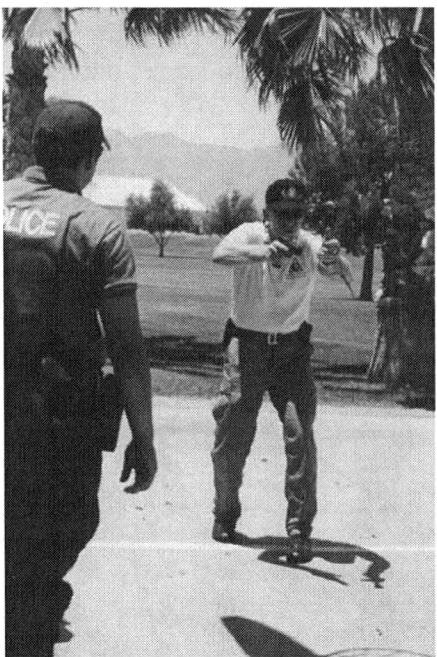

Images must be made dramatic, including movement with the imagery to create a full body experience to match what is being imagined.

Practice...Frequently

Just like physical skills, mental imagery can only be improved through practice. Spend time frequently working on imagery skills.

Integrate Imagery into Practice

There are countless opportunities during training to use imagery to help with operational skills...take advantage of these various opportunities. For example, correct techniques on the range visualizing real world conditions, add intensity and aggression to entry/clearing exercises, feeling fatigue and working through it.

TRAINER'S GUIDE

Teaching mental imagery may seem like a strange and uncomfortable task. How can you control or influence what your warriors imagine? Honestly, you can't! But with some patience and some guidance you can steer them in the right direction. In this section, I have provided you with a basic outline that should serve as a guide when working with your warrior's imagery skill.

Get their attention...

Like all other points of significance, you need to get your warriors' attention so they are motivated to use imagery. I have found that the following exercises can be beneficial in demonstrating to warriors the power of imagery.

Arm as an Iron Bar

Have warriors pair off. Instruct your warriors to stand facing each other about arm's length apart. Have warrior #1 rest an arm, palm up, on his partner's shoulder. Have warrior #2 take his hands and link them around warrior #1's extended arm, right above the elbow. Warrior #1 is then instructed to tighten his arm so as not to let warrior #2 bend it with his strength downward. This should be a fairly easy feat for warrior #2. Let each partner take a turn in both positions before moving on.

Next ask the warrior with his arm extended to imagine that starting from his shoulder his arm is a strong steel bar that extends through the wall. When this image is created, again have the other warrior push down on the arm. In most cases when the image of the steel bar is created the arm is much stronger in relation to the first attempt.

Explain to your warriors that they have just experienced the power of simple mental imagery. Just by imagining that their arm was an iron bar, they gained some strength. Now just imagine what can happen if this same skill is applied to other aspects of training.

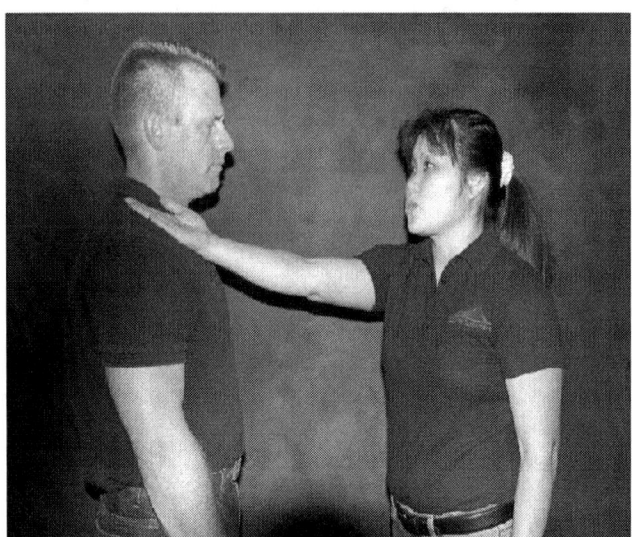

Arm as an iron bar — Working in pairs, have warriors stand facing each other about arm's length apart. Have warrior #1 rest an arm, palm up, on his partner's shoulder.

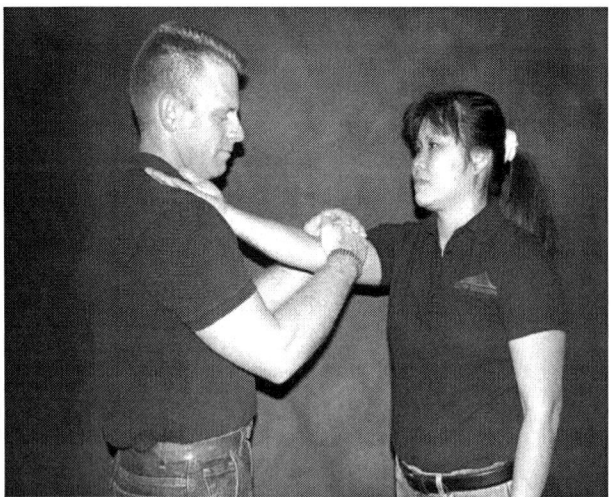

Arm as an iron bar — Have warrior #2 take his hands and link them around warrior #1's extended arm, right above the elbow.

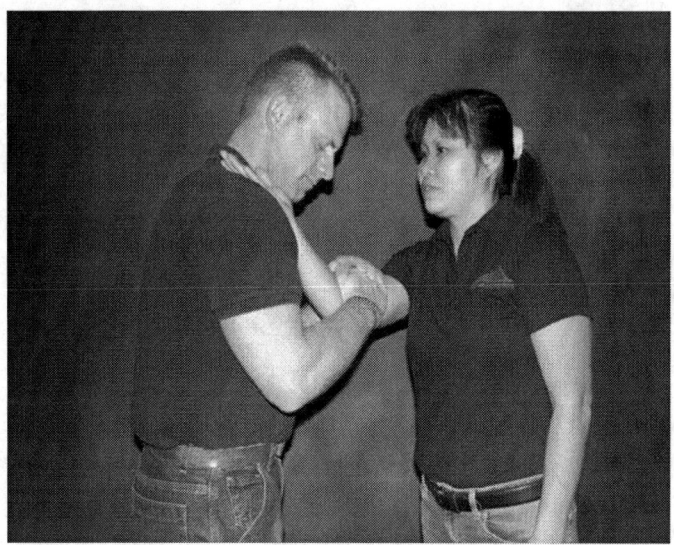

Arm as an iron bar — Warrior #1 is then instructed to tighten his arm so as not to let warrior #2 bend it with his strength downward.

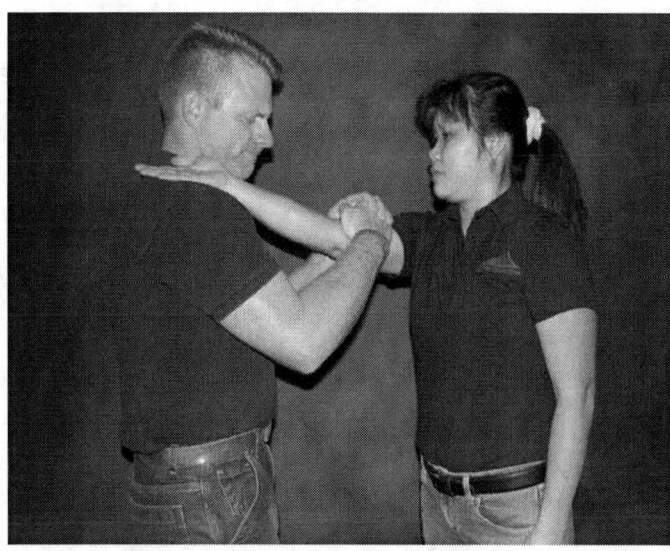

Arm as an iron bar — Have the warrior, with his arm extended, imagine that his arm is now a strong steel bar that extends through the wall behind his partner. With this image created, have the other warrior push down on the arm.

Bolt on a String

Give each of your warriors a string threaded through a large bolt. Have your warriors steady their elbows on a table or flat surface. Have them hold one of each of the two sides of the string in each hand, between the forefinger and thumb (so that the string forms a triangle, one side in each hand and the bolt hanging at the bottom). Instruct your warriors to imagine the bolt moving from side to side like a pendulum of a clock. Most warriors will experience some sort of movement in the bolt. Next, try to have the warriors move the bolt in a clockwise circle by just imagining it. You can also have them try counter-clockwise and front to back. In most cases warriors report movement in their bolts without purposely moving it.

To shed light on this exercise, tell your warriors that the subtle impulses sent from the brain to the arms and hands as a result of mental imagery and these muscle impulses are responsible for the movement in the bolt. Now, discuss how this concept applies to training and real world situations.

Teaching the Basics of Imagery

Take 5-10 minutes to review with your warriors the material presented at the beginning of this chapter. Place emphasis on how imagery can be used to improve performance and discuss tips to effective use of imagery.

Introductory imagery exercises (exercises 1 and 2)

We are now ready to have the warrior practice using imagery. Before asking your warriors to visualize themselves moving, acting and reacting there are several exercises you can use, to help them hone their imagery skills.

1. Have your warriors imagine an inanimate object related to their job, such as gloves, goggles, a baton, their firearm, etc. Talk them through the visualization asking them to imagine various aspects of the object such as color, size, feel, weight and shape. Speak

slowly and allow the warriors some time to draw a picture in their heads.

2. Instruct your warriors to imagine the area or facility they work or train in daily. Have them pay close attention to the smell of the air, the details of the facility, the lighting, and the feeling they have when they walk into the area or facility. Again, you are having your warriors imagine inanimate objects; this type of imagery will help them hone their imagery skills.

3. Think of any other inanimate/animate object for your warriors to visualize, their partner, magazine cover, the list is endless.

Basic imagery training exercises (exercises 2 and 4)

In the beginning, keep the imagery exercises simple. Do not try to immediately jump into a full speed run-through of events. Give your warriors a chance to sharpen their skills through less complex imagery training and then have them build up to real world simulations.

1. Spend some time allowing your warriors to imagine themselves working from both an internal and external perspective. Allow them to get comfortable with imagining their movements. You may want to try to incorporate some video at this point, so they can watch themselves working and also watch others working, who have good techniques or similar techniques.

2. If you are teaching a new skill, give your warriors a chance to incorporate the new skill into their imagery scripts. Spend some time imagining, as well as doing, the new skill.

Real world simulation (exercise 3)

Once your warriors have spent time working on basic imagery skills, they are now ready for a real world simulation. When first conducting a real world simulation imagery session, keep it short. Maybe only include the initial sequence of the event, depending on the complexity of the event. Keep in mind such details as pace, tempo, breathing and the overall feel of the environment.

Exercises to develop your mental imagery skills

The following is a preview of exercises included in this chapter to help develop imagery skills.

Exercises 1, 2, 3, 4 are for more seasoned and experienced warriors. They highlight many areas central to imagery, such as, incorporating all the senses, imagining your specific skills, using imagery in real world events and controlling the outcome of the images. Each of the worksheets should be used in conjunction with an imagery session.

Exercises 5 and 6 are designed for newer, less experienced warriors. They introduce the idea of creating images about training and the real world, then incorporating those images into daily imagery practice.

Sample imagery script
A sample imagery script has been included for your use. Consider this, like many other exercises, a facilitator for other imagery scripts. You are not required to use this one exclusively, change it to best suit your needs; this is only a suggested format to get you started with imagery.

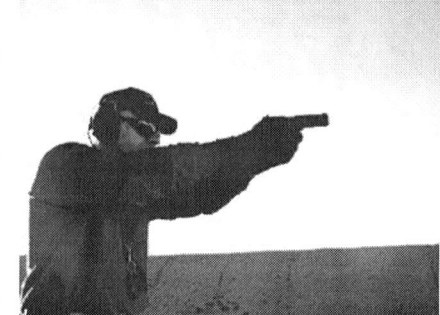

Developed skills in imagery can in fact turn goals into realities, seeing is believing and believing is winning!

At the end of the chapter is a section to aid in tracking imagery skill improvement.

IMAGERY - Exercise 1
Imagery sensory checklist

This is an exercise designed to assist you in beginning to integrate your senses into your imagery. As you create each of the following images in your mind, rate your ability to do so based on this scale.

0 = No Image   1 = Some Image   2 = Clear Image

_____ 1.   The room you are currently in.

_____ 2.   Your duty uniform.

_____ 3.   Tasting a juicy lemon.

_____ 4.   The sound of your alarm clock.

_____ 5.   The car you last drove.

_____ 6.   The feel at the end of a tour of duty.

_____ 7.   Performing calisthenics.

_____ 8.   Jumping into a cold pool of water.

_____ 9.   The sound of a noisy crowd.

_____ 10.   Feeling dry-mouthed and tired after a workout.

_____ 11.   The discomfort in your muscles during a grueling workout.

_____ 12.   The anticipation and anxiety of waiting to make an entry.

You may notice, as you review your scores, that certain senses produce clearer than others. This may provide direction for extra attention and practice—create your own images to test those senses with which you have the most difficulty.

IMAGERY - Exercise 2
Imaging your skills

As you refine your ability to image with all your senses, you want to begin using imagery to see yourself performing a skill in your specific area or occupation. Work through the progression at your own pace. For example, if you can't image yourself performing specific skills right now, keep working on your practice situation and movement imagery until they are very vivid and controllable before trying the specific skill section again.

Following these steps may make it easier to do this:

1. **Imagine that you are in the location or facility where you generally train.** Use your imaging skills to look around the training environment.

   - Feel the temperature of the facility
   - See what is generally around you: walls, equipment, teammates.
   - Imagine yourself in uniform, full duty or callout.

   What are some other things you can incorporate into this image from where you train?

2. **Incorporate some movement.** "Feel" yourself.

   - Walking around the area
   - Doing specific activities

   What are some other movements common to your area of specialty?

3. **Image yourself performing a skill in your specific occupation or area of specialty.** Start with a specific drill. Imagine yourself performing the drill correctly. Progress to imaging activities, each detail at a time.

   Are there some skills in your area of specialty you need to focus on?

What was easy and what was hard to image? Did you have a hard time using one sense or another? Could you see some things and not others? You'll want to practice more images that were harder to create.

IMAGERY - Exercise 3
Real world situation imagery

After mastering the exercises of the previous pages, you may find that you experience more "real life" emotion if you imagine yourself in a real world situation.

1. **Approach a place, through imagery, where you have recently worked, operated** or have vivid memories of an event. Allow yourself to experience the sensations that may accompany a real world experience for you—that is, if you typically get nervous or psyched up before work or a mission, allow yourself to feel those emotions.

   List some typical emotions or feelings that you experience before a specific event.

2. **Imagine yourself at varying times before the event.** Making it as real and vivid as possible. If you typically have a pre-event routine, imagine yourself following the steps of that routine up to the point where you are initiating the event. Remember to use all your senses.

   Write down what you typically do before an event.

3. **Real world time:** Imagine yourself in an actual real world situation, doing what you would typically do, with your typical emotional and physical reactions.

   — At the beginning and throughout the event, **I feel**:

   — At the beginning and throughout the event, **I do:**

   — At the beginning and throughout the event, **I think:**

   — At the beginning and throughout the event, **I see:**

IMAGERY - Exercise 4
Controlling outcome

The key to imagery as a performance enhancement tool is not just to make vivid images, but ones that **you** can control—making happen what you want to have happen.

Go back to exercise 33, but decide beforehand how you **want** to be feeling and saying to yourself before you approach the event site. Repeat each step, but with the addition of changes that reflect those changed thoughts and feelings.

1. **Approach a place, through imagery, where you have recently operated,** or have vivid memories of an event.

   How I **want** to be feeling:

   What I **want** to be saying to myself:

2. **Imagine yourself at varying times before an event.**

   How I **want** to be feeling:

   What I **want** to be saying to myself:

3. **During the event.**

   How I **want** to be feeling:

   What I **want** to be saying to myself:

If this is a difficult change to make, you may find yourself lapsing back to images of what typically happens rather than what you wanted to happen. If this happens, "rewind" or repeat the image experience until you are able to control it. It is counterproductive to image scenes that you cannot control or that lead to undesirable outcomes.

IMAGERY - Exercise 5
News Flash

Imagine that there is a news reporter at your next event. You have worked hard and performed great. Before you can relax, the reporter runs to meet you and asks you about the event. Create the news headline that the reporter will run on the front page.

Headline:

News Report:

IMAGERY - Exercise 6

Act like...

Oftentimes imagining a specific image (object, animal, person) can aid in your creation of images. You've probably heard your trainer or leader say something like, "Take off like a bullet!" "Swim like a fish," or "Slice the pie." In the following spaces provided, pick a skill you are working on in training and choose an image to pair with that skill.

Skill:

Image:

How this image will help:

Skill

Image:

How this image will help:

Skill:

Image:

How this image will help:

Sample Imagery Script

As you and your team make an initial approach to the door of a suspect residence, you immediately recognize the familiar smell of sweat and one of your teammate's cigarettes...You scan the environment...Taking in the overall layout of the residence and everyone present...You notice the sounds of yourself and your team...Voices under breath and rapid breathing...The sound of the ground under your feet...The periodic sound of a car passing on the road behind the residence.

You imagine yourself getting ready to make entry...Getting in your position in the stack...Getting in position immediately behind the man to your front...Going over last minute details in your head...This is your time to shine...You're prepared for this event and you are feeling mentally strong.

The team leader begins the count down for entry...Imagine yourself, weapon at the outboard...Your head down, knees flexed...At the signal, you move...A strong powerful purposeful movement into the enclosure...You feel air pass your skin...The sound of movement is all around you.

Every step you feel strong...Moving through the portal into the enclosure...You're moving at a strong and steady tempo...You're covering your areas of responsibility...You can see your teammates off to your sides...You see them but you don't break from your responsibilities...You glide through the enclosure, room to room...You come around a corner into a new, unsecured room...You complete the turn into the room...You come face to face with your suspect...He is in your sector...You order him down...He complies.

As you begin your secondary checks, you are still feeling strong and focused...You've trained hard for moments like this...You continue through the structure and account for your men and your gear...You breathe...You're thinking...You're lucid...You clear the structure, you walk with great poise and purpose...You realize you have achieved your goal, your mission...You regain awareness of those things outside of your mission...You become aware of the feelings of excitement and

accomplishment...Pride builds inside you...You have succeeded...
You are a winner!

How to Track Imagery Skill Improvement

There are a number of ways to measure your imagery skill
development. The most basic is to track the time you practice
each day. As described earlier in this book, keeping log books of
both training and real world events are important; add a section
for imagery to your log books.

Another possibility for tracking improvement includes seeing
how long you can consistently hold an image, by timing yourself
throughout an imagery session. Imagery takes a lot of concentration, and you may find that you cannot hold an image for
very long at first, but you can develop this part of your skill with
consistent effort.

Good luck...Train to win!

Chapter Five

SELF-TALK: WARRIOR, COACH THYSELF

"It is fatal to enter any war without the will to win it."
— Douglas MacArthur

What Is Self-talk?

Self-talk is the sum total of all purposeful and random thoughts that can run through an individual's mind. It includes all things said internally and aloud. Self-talk can be positive, it can tell a warrior what to do, where and when to focus, and it can serve to motivate ("I can do it!"). Unfortunately, self-talk can also be negative ("I can't!"), pessimistic, and destructively critical. Negative self-talk does nothing to help performance and for the most part, it causes severe problems in performance. In our line of work they are potentially life-threatening problems. Recognize that negative self-talk will occur, regardless of who you are, you're still human; the key is not to dwell on negatives, rather focus on the positives.

When Self-talk Goes Bad

There are consistent self-talk errors that we, as humans, make that provide a negative influence on our performance, they are listed in the following passages. As you read them I am quite sure you'll recognize having experienced a few of them.

Focusing on the Past or on the Future

"I screwed up the last time we did this." "I can't believe I did so badly." Failing to let go of mistakes or poor performance takes thoughts and focus away from where they need to be—focused on things at hand!

Focusing on Weaknesses

To improve performance for critical situations, it is necessary to identify and correct weaknesses, but this correction should occur in training only. During actual operational environments, dwelling on shortcomings will quickly erode confidence. Ideally, the real world is where warriors should focus on strengths as a warrior by emphasizing positive thoughts.

Focusing Solely on the Outcome

"I have to win it all!" "I have to make it through selection!" Thoughts like these direct individuals to the outcome or the end result of a process, a process that they have little control over. What we as warriors do have control over is immediate performance in any given situation. Self-talk should be directed towards the steps in the process, the things that need to be done to succeed, trusting that the outcome will be there.

Focusing on Uncontrollable Factors

"I hate training when it rains." "I never shoot well when I am on the end target." These are pure wastes of valuable mental energy and time. Not only are these out of our control, but they distract us from things of importance. Keep thoughts on controllable factors.

Demanding Perfection

"I better kick ass!" "My execution must be perfect." Warriors train their physical skills for years, trying to achieve perfect performance. It is appropriate to work towards perfection, but unrealistic to expect a perfect performance in every situation.

Putting an End to Negative Self-talk

Just like physical skills that warriors train on a regular basis, controlling self-talk is also a skill. For some warriors who have fallen into a pattern of negative, defeating self-talk, learning to gain control can be hard. Negative internal talk is something warriors are often no longer aware of, it seems to happen automatically. Therefore before changing self-talk, it is necessary to take a step back and become aware of what is being said. It is necessary to identify both beneficial thoughts and harmful thoughts. Once this is accomplished it is important to make a conscious effort to purposely include those thoughts that seem to help performance.

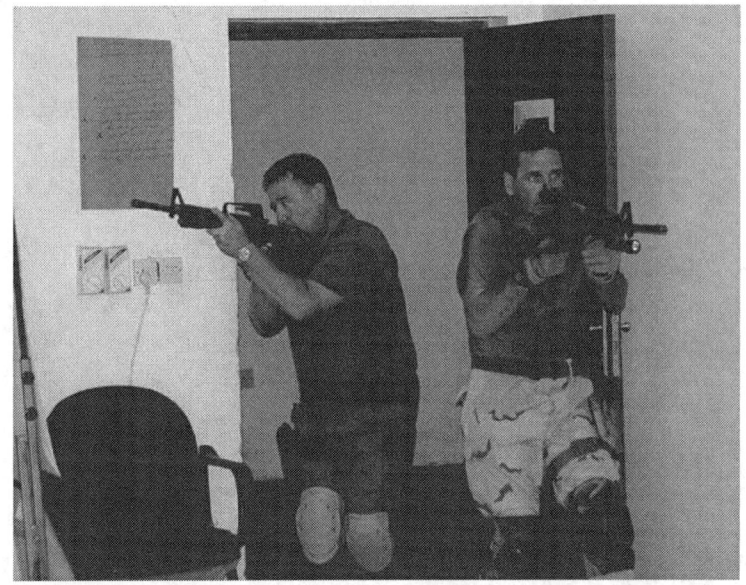

Dwelling on negative self-talk causes severe problems in performance, potentially life-threatening problems.

Thought stopping is the most common technique used to introduce positive thoughts and eliminate negative thoughts.

1. Become Aware of Self-talk

As previously noted, the first step in gaining control of self-talk is by increasing awareness of what warriors tend to say to themselves both in training and in operational situations, as well as the typical situations where these thoughts occur.

For example, it may be that at the beginning of a training event, a warrior feels strong, tending to have positive, confident thoughts. But, toward the culmination of the event, when the warrior feels fatigued, he begins to question his ability.

2. Stop the Negative

Once negative self-talk is identified, the warrior needs to learn to "knock it off!" This, of course, is much easier said than done! Saying "knock it off!" or visualizing a stop sign are good positive cues to help halt negative thoughts.

3. Replace with Positive

Imagine that the mind is like a bowl—if it is filled to the brim with positive thoughts, there will be no room for negative self-talk. Warriors need to identify positive self-talk in advance and replace the negative thoughts with identified positive ones.

4. Practice Thought-stopping

A final step is to practice, practice, practice stopping and replacing negative talk. For awhile, warriors will need to be very conscious of their internal self-talk as the thought-stopping technique will not occur automatically. With enough practice, positive self-talk will become second nature. Exercise 1 will take warriors step by step through the technique of thought-stopping. Complete the exercise several times to take into account all the situations in which negative self-talk initiates.

Additional tips

Tell Yourself What You Can do...

Here is a quick exercise...Picture your home in your mind. See the surroundings. Now, the challenge is for you to tell yourself to NOT think about a large piece of rotting meat sitting in the middle of your living room and to actually NOT think about it. Chances are the first thing that popped into your head was thoughts of the rotting meat.

What typically happens when an individual tells himself not to do something like, "don't screw up," "don't look," and "don't miss the target," the individual immediately thinks about what they are NOT supposed to do or think and oftentimes they actually do those very things. A more effective strategy is to direct self-talk so you are telling yourself what to do rather than what not to do.

Plant Positives

Instead of waiting until self-talk starts spiraling out of control, purposefully plant positive thoughts and comments in your mind so there is no room for negatives.

Develop an Event Self-talk Plan

Another helpful technique that promotes beneficial self-talk is related to real-world event preparation (exercise 3). Just as a warrior develops an operational event plan or strategy and reviews this using mental rehearsal, he can also develop an operational event self-talk plan. Warriors should prepare in advance what they want to say to themselves and what needs to be reinforced in order to perform their best; part of any real world event preparation should involve mentally rehearsing this strategy until it becomes habit.

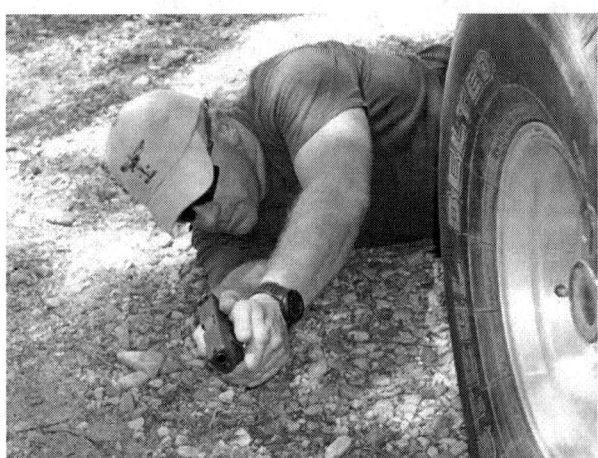

By identifying positive self-talk in advance of an incident, replacing the negative thoughts with identified positive thoughts can end negative thoughts.

```
                    TRAINER'S GUIDE
```

Grab Their Attention...

Although everyone talks to themselves at one time or another, some individuals may not be aware of what they say to themselves. The following exercise is a great way to help your warriors become more aware of what they say to themselves.

Would You Say it to Your Partner?

At the beginning of your self-talk session hand out exercise 4 and a pen or pencil. Ask your warriors to think of a time during a training session or even a real world event where they made a big mistake. Then ask them to remember what they said to themselves in that situation. Have them write it down in the top box of exercise 4.

At this point instruct your warriors to pair off. Have them turn to their partner and read the self-talk they wrote on their sheets out loud to their partner with feeling, similar to the way they would have said it to themselves.

Now, turn the focus of the exercise from a negative to a positive. Have your warriors re-phrase their original self-talk into a more positive manner in the bottom box of exercise 4. Again ask them to share this statement with their partner for more feedback.

Tips for Training Self-talk

- Begin with the previously described exercise. Grab your warriors' attention and get them thinking about the meaning of the phrase "Self-talk."
- Ask your warriors to define self-talk. Spend some time covering the common self-talk errors and give examples in each situation. Have your warriors consider their behavior in each of these situations.
- Introduce the steps to changing negative self-talk and spend some time on the exercises included at the end of this chapter.
- For a long-term plan, have your warriors create a self-talk section in their training logbooks. Help them monitor

their own self-talk and assist them in changing their self-talk behavior.

Self-talk Exercises

The following is a description of exercises designed both to identify what warriors say to themselves and how they say it. Feel free to pick and choose the exercises that best suit you and your warriors.

Exercise 1 is a thought-stoppage exercise. Sometimes, as warriors are talking to themselves, they get into a habit of using negative words and phrases. This exercise will help warriors to stop those negative thoughts and come up with new positive ones.

Exercise 2 is designed for warriors to recognize what they are saying to themselves and how to change those thoughts from negative ones to positive ones.

Exercise 3 teaches warriors how to use cue words in developing an event plan. Developing an event plan of positive cue words can help to control self-talk. If you already know what you are going to say during specific points of an event, the chances of negative thoughts entering your mind can be decreased.

Exercise 4 is the worksheet designed to accompany the initial "Grab their attention..." exercise.

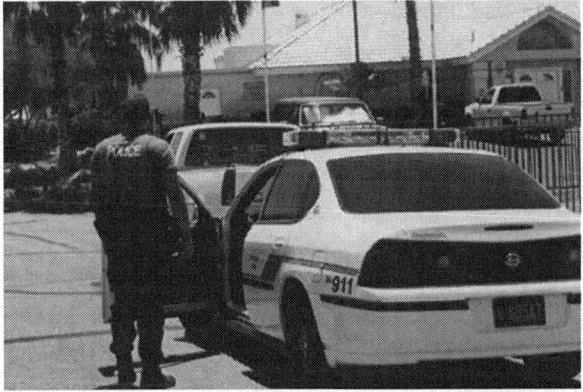

The use of cue words is crucial in developing an event plan and to control self-talk. Knowing what you are going to say during an event limits the chances of negative thoughts entering your mind.

SELF-TALK - Exercise 1
Thought-stopping

Example: Rich is a perfectionist. Every time he trains he expects not only to be better than his teammates, but also to have absolute perfect form and technique. After all, he is training harder than anyone else, putting in extra time and energy, he has sacrificed a lot. Rich doesn't just want to be proficient, but believes he has to and should flawlessly every time. Over time, Rich realized that such thoughts were harmful to overall performance so he started working on controlling his overly demanding self-talk. What follows is an example of a "Thought-Stopping" form that Rich has completed and has been implementing in training and in real world situations.

---

1. SITUATION:

During pre-event preparation, I am very demanding of myself. This seems to put a lot of pressure on me and causes me to get tense and anxious knowing I have to perform flawlessly.

2. NEGATIVE STATEMENT:

"I have to be perfect!" "I can make no mistakes!" "Zero defects!"

3. STOPPING THE NEGATIVE THOUGHT:

"Knock it off, Rich!" (I say this to myself while taking a slow, deep breath and focusing on relaxing.)

4. POSITIVE REPLACEMENT:

"Do your best!" "Work hard!" "Watch your areas of responsibility." "Stay alert, stay alive!" (Self-talk will be focused on what I need to do to perform my best.)

Go on to next page and fill out your own "Thought-Stopping Form."

SELF-TALK - Exercise 1a
Thought-stopping

1. DESCRIBE A SITUATION IN WHICH YOU OFTEN TEND TO
   THINK/TALK NEGATIVELY TO YOURSELF:

2. IDENTIFY THE NEGATIVE STATEMENT YOU SAY TO
   YOURSELF:

3. IDENTIFY WORDS OR THOUGHTS YOU CAN USE TO HELP
   YOU STOP THE NEGATIVE THOUGHT:

4. LIST POSITIVE, BENEFICIAL STATEMENTS YOU CAN USE
   TO REPLACE NEGATIVE HARMFUL THOUGHTS. THESE
   SHOULD BE MEANINGFUL TO YOU:

5. PRACTICE! PRACTICE! PRACTICE THIS TECHNIQUE WHILE
   TRAINING.

SELF-TALK - Exercise 2
Changing negative thoughts to positive

Identify the negative and positive thoughts that you have in training, before a real world event and even before and after an event. Make sure you examine the differences carefully. If you do not have any positive thoughts, work on changing your negative thoughts into positive ones.

THOUGHTS I HAVE IN TRAINING...	
NEGATIVE	POSITIVE

THOUGHTS I HAVE IN REAL-WORLD/OPERATIONAL EVENTS...	
NEGATIVE	POSITIVE

THOUGHTS I HAVE BEFORE & AFTER A REAL-WORLD / OPERATIONAL EVENT...	
NEGATIVE	POSITIVE

SELF-TALK - Exercise 3
Event plan

In the table provided include positive cue words (such as push, harder, go, move, steady, etc)

SPECIFIC POINTS BEFORE,	CUE WORDS
ONE HOUR BEFORE THE EVENT	
10 MINUTES BEFORE THE EVENT	
EVENT INITIATION	
MIDWAY THROUGH THE EVENT	
NEAR EVENT TERMINATION	
EVENT TERMINATION	
ONE HOUR FOLLOWING EVENT	

SELF-TALK - Exercise 4
Get their attention...

THINK ABOUT THE LAST TIME YOU MADE A SUBSTANTIAL
MISTAKE DURING TRAINING OR A REAL-WORLD EVENT.

WHAT DID YOU SAY TO YOURSELF?

RESTATE WHAT YOU SAID TO YOURSELF IN A POSITIVE &
PRODUCTIVE FORMAT.

NOW WHAT WOULD YOU SAY?

Chapter Six

SELF-CONFIDENCE: KNOWING AND BELIEVING IN YOUR OWN ABILITIES

"This is the law of the Yukon, that only the strong shall thrive; that surely the weak shall perish, and only the fit survive."
— Robert W. Service

What is Self-confidence?

I f I were to ask you to picture in your mind a strong, confident warrior, how would you describe this person? Descriptions typically used include: head up, alert, shoulders back, talks about effective skills, manages anxiety, unfazed by stress, etc. While these descriptions may be accurate, a characteristic of a confident warrior that you can't see is **TRUST**—inner trust or conviction in their ability to operate regardless of the external environment. Over two decades ago when I was in basic training, my Drill Sergeant would frequently say wonderfully meaningful phrases, in between periods of motivational training (a PC way of saying grueling, ass-kicking, morale-breaking, physical training). One of the things he would say that has stuck with me my entire life was, "Discipline, the overwhelming obedience to orders!" "Regardless of whether those orders were given to you or you gave them to yourself!" "The ability to follow those orders, regardless of minor discomforts like: heat, cold, fatigue and pain!" This concept resonates the essence of this section of the book...Confidence and the belief in yourself. The ability to overlook distractions in critical environments and knowing that you can win regardless of the odds. Wow! Powerful words, God bless you, SFC Steven Terrell, wherever you are!

Essentially, self-confidence is the belief in one's ability to succeed. When your trainer or team leader tells you what drills to perform, confidence is the belief that you can complete the drills to standard, regardless of the level of complexity. When you are standing in a stack positioned at someone's front door for the first time, getting ready to breach and clear the enclosure,

133

confidence is the belief in your ability to operate up to your capabilities (as you have demonstrated throughout training). Research on the elite suggests that a high level of confidence, as well as the ability to maintain that high level over time, is a critical factor in their performance. The challenge is in figuring out how this skill/characteristic can be developed in warriors from all career fields.

Contrary to what most people think, people who have high self-confidence sometimes doubt themselves or their abilities; elite athletes report feelings of apprehension and pressure prior to competition, but still perform well. So being confident does not mean the total absence of negative feelings. Rather, self-confident individuals believe in their ability to perform well despite feelings such as apprehension or doubt. For example, when training has been going poorly or when performances are below expectation, confident warriors still believe in their ability to perform well. This is not an easy task!

The Value of Being a Confident Warrior

As discussed, high self-confidence is a characteristic that we tend to see and expect in those with elite status. To convince you that working to develop and control self-confidence is critical, I am going to describe positive characteristics that are associated with high confidence. To increase your self-confidence try thinking and behaving this way:

Confident Warriors Unfailingly Work Hard, Practice Hard and Play Hard

Confident warriors know that much of their confidence is developed through experiencing success. They have learned to work on the controllable factors in training and rehearsals that can be developed to help them enhance their abilities (cultivating success). They know that to be confident when they roll on real world events, they have to put in the work!

Confident Warriors Focus on Controllable Factors

Instead of spending time griping and stressing about what they cannot do or might not be able to do, or otherwise doubting themselves, confident warriors are more able to focus on tasks at hand. While the doubt and concern they experience is real, they know that what is most advantageous is to focus on what they **CAN** do.

Confident Warriors Try Even Harder When They Don't Reach Their Goals

One significant difference between more and less confident operators is how each group interprets "failure." Confident individuals are more likely to view failure as a result of a lack of effort, preparation, concentration, skill execution, or other factors they have the ability to change. On the other hand, individuals who are less confident view failure as a lack of ability, something they have less ability to change.

Confident Operators Commit to Winning

You have likely heard the comments of "doing it to win" and "doing it not to lose." While these two might sound similar, they are both significantly different. Doing any project to win means the individual is not afraid to take chances and take control of a situation. When an individual commits to "not to lose" the focus is on the negative and is reactive as opposed to proactive behavior. Confident warriors always do it to win!

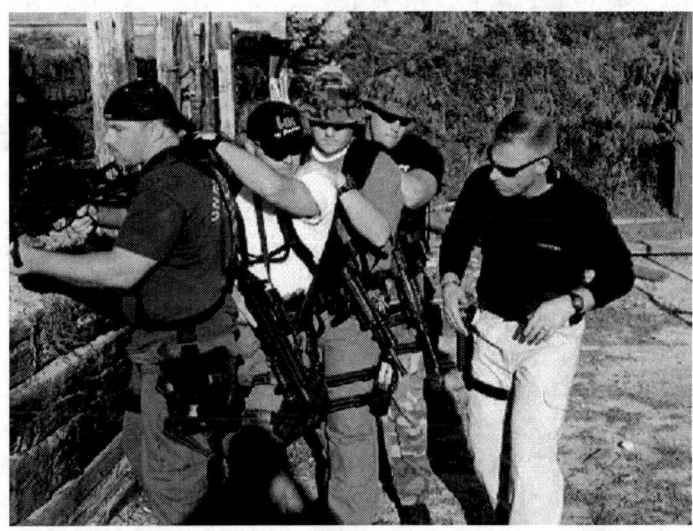

When warriors refuse to lose, the focus is on positive pro-active performance, confident warriors always do it to win!

Confident Warriors Control Their Emotions

Individuals with high self-confidence are better able to recoil from adversity (like poor qualification scores or a bad evaluation) than those individuals who are less confident. Instead of getting angry, upset, depressed, or pessimistic, confident warriors control these potentially catastrophic emotions. Warriors who are confident in themselves and their abilities have a "can do" and "never quit" attitude, viewing situations where things go against them as challenges, as opposed to immovable barriers.

Improving Self-confidence

It is important that all warriors and trainers recognize that success breeds confidence. Because confidence is so critical to performance, especially performance under high duress circumstances, a tremendous amount of research has looked at how confidence is developed and we have found that the best way to develop confidence is through performance accomplishments; in other words, through success. This success can be found in both practice and under operational conditions. To build confidence, one can recall past successes—visualizing images and feelings of success, which can also serve as validation that that individual "Can do it!" And, as discussed in following passages, one can create success. The challenge lies when operational successes are few and far between.

It is critical to build success into each and every training event. It was discussed that success breeds confidence, which leads one to suggest that you need to find "success" on a consistent basis. You are doing good things all the time in training; now, you need to be purposeful about making note of all successes because it is these daily successes that you can carry with you, daily at work to enhance your belief that you really are ready to win, regardless of the circumstances. One way to do this is by keeping a log of successes, where you record daily successes. Another strategy is to establish a goal setting system (refer to the chapter on goal setting). By setting goals and achieving them you are in essence structuring success into your training environment.

Observing others and modeling their successes is another viable strategy. While not as powerful as successfully performing the skill or behavior yourself, watching others who are similar to you experience success has been found to be another strategy to enhancing confidence. For example, watching a teammate, whom you train with regularly, move swiftly through an obstacle course, can enhance your confidence in your ability to also move as swiftly. Or, watching a video of a well executed technique, then using imagery to see yourself executing the technique can also build confidence in your ability to actually execute the technique.

Utilizing self-talk to establish confidence is another good tool. Confidence means thinking that you can and will achieve your goals. Persuade yourself, through self-talk, that you are capable, you can perform with great skill, you will execute your training and/or operational strategy, and you can make all the standards required. Monitor what you say to yourself and make sure your internal talk is instructional and motivational, in lieu of being unbelieving and negative (refer to the chapter on self-talk).

A general attitude of confidence, and acting confidently, is paramount. Your thoughts, feelings, and behaviors are all related—if you act confidently, this should enhance your feelings of confidence. This is truly important when you begin to lose confidence. Put a confident front on during operational settings by keeping your head high—even after a less than stellar performance. Behave with confidence (remember, head up, bounce to your step, focus on controllable factors) to trigger your confident mindset.

Recovering Confidence When Things Are Going less than Perfect

When things are flowing, reaction and response times drop, your team leader tells you how sharp you look (you know this is not patronage, because you feel it, too.)…confidence seems to ooze from every pore. You're performing well in training and you have good reason to be confident in your ability to perform. During rough times, performance heads into a slump when you don't feel right inside… these are times when it is most challenging to remain confident. What can you do to still believe in your abilities when your "abilities" seem to have left you?

Unfortunately, there is no simple answer. It is truly difficult to believe in an ability to perform well when you aren't performing well. However, I can offer a few strategies and suggestions to help you recover your confidence when things are going less than perfect.

Focus on Achievable Goals

In lieu of setting a goal to perform, which may or may not always be a realistic goal based on the moment, focus on a goal that is challenging yet immediately realistic. For example, an immediate goal may be to cut your time in a particular speed shooting drill or to breach an exterior door quickly and smoothly.

Re-create Past Successes

Go back, in your mind, to a previous training evolution or successful event. Recall how you felt and what you said to yourself and how you focused when training or operating. Try to re-create that. Set the stage for success. While a multitude of factors affect performance, your attitude and your thoughts have tremendous influence. Make every effort to re-create the mental environment that has proven beneficial.

Carry Positives With You

When you're not performing optimally, there is a tendency to be attuned to negatives, a natural human inclination to drift towards great negativity; to focus on all negative things that further confirm you are not operating so well. For example, a warrior who is struggling will get out of practice and remember only the negative feelings felt during the last training session. You need to force yourself to acknowledge the positives—the good things that occurred, such as improvements in techniques or feeling better than the day before. These positives should go with you to training sessions and certainly into the field.

Develop a Stick-to-it Plan

Prior to your involvement in a new, high training demand, endeavor, figure out how you are going to execute the demands of training and how you need to be, physically and mentally, to operate well. "Plant" the things you want to say to yourself, decide how you are going to focus before and during both training and real world situations, and commit to doing it. Too often, warriors get distracted by environmental things and allow extraneous thoughts and feelings to enter into their minds (thoughts that can be detrimental to confidence). Develop a plan in advance; one that is conducive to confident feelings.

Be Patient

Accept that your confidence will not rebound in the blink of an eye. It is undoubtedly going to take perseverance, persistence, and patience on your part to cultivate an ability to maintain high confidence, regardless of the environment.

TRAINER'S GUIDE

- Begin having your warriors define what self-confidence means to them. Encourage them to give examples of when they feel high and low self-confidence.
- Explain the difference between too much, too little and just right self-confidence.
- Tell your warriors about the benefits of increasing their self-confidence.
- Use one of the exercises of your choice to help your warriors become aware of their self-confidence.
- Instruct your warriors on ways to improve their self-confidence.

Whether you know it or not, you can influence your warriors' self-confidence. Warriors look to their supervisors, their peers, and their trainers for feedback and for approval. Do not take your job lightly, what you say to your warriors and the tone of voice and words you use will greatly influence their perceptions of themselves.

When correcting mistakes and giving feedback, use a "sandwich" type technique—meaning try to sandwich the critique between two positive comments. Start by relaying a positive comment, follow that by a correction (what they should do) and end with encouragement and optimism.

Self-confidence Exercises

The following are some ideas of ways for warriors to develop their own sense of self-confidence.

Exercise 1 is developed to encourage warriors to brainstorm about their positive abilities and attributes. This exercise can be used for both newer and more seasoned warriors.

Exercise 2 emphasizes using mental imagery as a means of increasing self-confidence.

Exercise 3 suggests that the warriors begin keeping a success log. A success log is a place where warriors are encouraged to write down things that they do well, both in and outside of training or work. This again will help raise the warriors' awareness to their personal accomplishments.

Exercise 4 helps warriors create their own personal affirmations. Personal affirmations serve to remind warriors of their strengths or the behaviors they want to develop into strengths.

SELF-CONFIDENCE - Exercise 1
Raise Self-confidence Awareness

As a way to gain thinking about self-confidence in your specific pursuit, the first step is to identify your abilities and other positive attributes. Complete the following statements with a variety of different skills and attributes, using examples from both work and outside of work. This activity highlights the many talents you possess. Concentrate more on developing this list rather than spending time worrying about what you can't do.

1. SOMETHING I DO WELL IN MY FIELD OF:_____

2. SOMETHING I DO EVEN BETTER IN MY FIELD OF: _____

3. MY GREATEST STRENGTH AS A WARRIOR IS: _____

4. I AM PROUD THAT I: _____

5. MY GREATEST STRENGTH AS AN INDIVIDUAL IS: _____

6. I CAN HELP MY TEAMMATES TO: _____

7. I HAVE POWER TO: _____

8. I WAS ABLE TO DECIDE TO: _____

9. I'M NOT AFRAID TO: _____

10. I WANT TO BE STRONG ENOUGH TO: _____

11. SOMETHING I CAN DO NOW THAT I COULDN'T IN THE PAST IS: _____

12. I HAVE ACCOMPLISHED: _____

13. IF I WANT TO, I CAN: _____

14. MY GREATEST ACHIEVEMENT IS: _____

SELF-CONFIDENCE - Exercise 2
Building through the past

Consistent good performances directly and positively impact self-confidence. So it stands to reason that the more consistently good performances you can have, the more likely they will be to feed an individual's self-confidence. This is especially true for warriors who know they have the ability, but have trouble building their confidence to believe that their ability will transfer to different situations.

REMEMBER BACK TO YOUR BEST PERFORMANCE EVER AND ANSWER
THE QUESTIONS PERTAINING TO THAT EVENT.

WHAT DID YOU EAT THE NIGHT BEFORE?

HOW MANY HOURS OF SLEEP DID YOU GET THE NIGHT BEFORE?

WHAT TIME DID YOU WAKE UP? HOW MANY HOURS WAS IT BEFORE THE EVENT?

WHAT DID YOU EAT FOR BREAKFAST?

WHAT DID YOU DO PRIOR TO THE EVENT?

HOW DID YOU FEEL THE NIGHT BEFORE THE EVENT?

HOW DID YOU FEEL DURING THE EVENT?

WHAT DID YOU DO IMMEDIATELY AFTER THE EVENT?

NOW THAT YOU'VE REFLECTED ON ALL OF THESE THOUGHTS, FEELINGS AND ACTIONS,
TRY TO INCORPORATE THEM INTO YOUR NEXT EVENT. BY RECOGNIZING WHAT YOU DID
THE LAST TIME YOU WERE SUCCESSFUL AND INCORPORATING IT INTO YOUR
NEXT EVENT, YOU CAN BEGIN TO PRACTICE SUCCESS ON A REGULAR BASIS.

SELF-CONFIDENCE - Exercise 3
Success Log

Some warriors have difficulty recalling previous performance or successes to use in their confidence building. Sometimes this is due to a simple lack of awareness—the warrior has never had to "tune in" to this before and may need to learn to pay better attention to his or her performances. Often, especially for perfectionist, high-achieving warriors, it has become easier for them to pay attention to their mistakes as opposed to good things that have happened in practice.

To help you begin to redirect your focus to include the awareness of your successes, the "success log" has been developed. The idea is simple. After each training session and every real-world event, you must write down three things you did correctly or successfully. At first, some warriors find the adjustment in focus a little hard since being critical and focusing on mistakes has been their habit for some time. Filling in your success log on a regular basis can assist with seeing the whole of a performance—both good and bad—and will provide you with much more confidence-building material.

EXAMPLE:

TRAINING DAY

1. ARRIVED ON TIME AND PREPARED FOR TRAINING

2. I WAS ABLE TO MAINTAIN GOOD FORM AND SAFETY THROUGH ALL LIVE FIRE DRILLS

3. I QUALIFIED 3 POINTS HIGHER THAN THE LAST QUALIFICATION

As you can see from the example, you can begin with positives that may not be directly related to your performance.

SELF-CONFIDENCE - Exercise 4
Affirmations

Affirmations can be an extremely strong tool to help build self-confidence. An affirmation is a statement that refers to something that is true or that warriors can use to direct their thoughts and behaviors in positive ways. They can be used to redirect negative thoughts. Often people feel that when they use affirmations they are deceiving themselves. However it is better to think of affirmations as a sense of direction, not deception.

THERE ARE FIVE CRITERIA TO KEEP IN MIND WHEN DEVELOPING YOUR OWN AFFIRMATIONS

1. BE POSITIVE

2. WRITE IT PRESENT TENSE

3. BE SHORT AND CONCISE

4. TRY TO MAKE IT RHYME, FOR EASE OF REMEMBRANCE

5. BE CONSCIENTIOUS, TRY TO RECITE YOUR AFFIRMATION AT LEAST ONCE A DAY

EXAMPLES OF AFFIRMATION USED TO BOOST CONFIDENCE:

"I AM SWIFT AND SURE AS I MOVE THROUGH AN ENCLOSURE"

"I AM A WINNER"

"I AM STRONG AND READY TO GO"

"I WILL NEVER QUIT"

Chapter Seven

CONCENTRATION: FOCUS ON THE RIGHT THING

"The first and the best victory is to conquer self."
— Plato

Concentrate! Keep your head in the game! Stay focused! You've probably heard this somewhere before. The ability to obtain and maintain concentration while immersed in the stress and anxiety of training and real world events is key to optimum performance, probably more so than any other element. If you lose your focus to a dedicated opponent, giving way to nagging self-doubt, you're not just battling him, but also battling yourself. Although we may not always be able to eliminate distractions, successful warriors take control of their performance by blocking out unnecessary distractions while observing and responding to important cues.

Top performance in high demand, high stress situations involves attending to the most appropriate portions of a task or selective attention. This refers to the process by which relevant information is selected for attention and irrelevant information is ignored or purged. As an example, consider a baseball game with a batter waiting at home plate for the pitch. As the pitch is released, the batter is more likely to focus on the rotation of the ball than the size of the crowd in the stands. Why? Because identifying the pitch is a fundamental aspect of the game and hitting the ball, whereas the size of the crowd is not. This focus or emphasis on concentration is what lets a batter decide on whether or not to swing at a 90 MPH fast ball, giving him the ability to make that decision in the .45 seconds it takes for that ball to make it from the pitcher's hand to the catcher's glove. The process of selection is essential, given the amount of information that the warrior is faced with. In conflict, selective attention to relevant information and active avoidance of irrelevant information is pivotal to peak performance. Thus, cultivating concentration skills is critical.

What is Concentration?

Concentration is paying attention to the right thing at the right time. It is the ability to attend to relevant factors and disregard irrelevant factors. This is not an easy task given all the internal and external factors that are present in training and in the real world. As you are in hot pursuit on a crowded highway, where are you focused? While waiting for the next overt action of the perpetrator, how is your mind occupied? When you are at the end of the pursuit, what are you focusing on? What things break your concentration? By identifying the attentional demands of your activity, you can direct your focus more effectively. Chance favors only the prepared mind. Prepare to excel by preparing to concentrate **(training to win)**.

Figuring out What to Focus on

A primary challenge related to effective concentration is figuring out the right and relevant factors to attend to in various training and real world situations. While knowing where to focus is no guarantee of being able to concentrate effectively, it is a step in the right direction. In determining where to focus, it makes innate sense to place mental energy on things that one can control. Rather than focusing on what an opponent is doing (which you can't control), it is more productive to focus on what you can control...your own performance.

Controlling the Controllable Things

An initial strategy to aid in figuring out where to focus is to distinguish between controllable and uncontrollable factors. In fact, ineffective concentration can often be traced to focusing on uncontrollable variables. For example:

- Do you ever fall into the trap of focusing on mistakes? No one is perfect. In the heat of action or in the middle of training, mistakes happen. If you allow yourself to be distracted by a mistake and dwell on it, you are in fact creating a lapse in concentration. Let the mistake go, it cannot be changed. Move past it and on to the next event, and focus your attention on the present, on what you can control.

- Do you get caught focusing too far in the future? Do you play the "What if" game? "What if I screw up?" "What if I lose?" Concentrating on future events also negatively affects concentration. By focusing on the mistakes that may be made in the future, poor performance is actually more likely to happen. Once again try to focus on the present, the here and now—this is what you control!

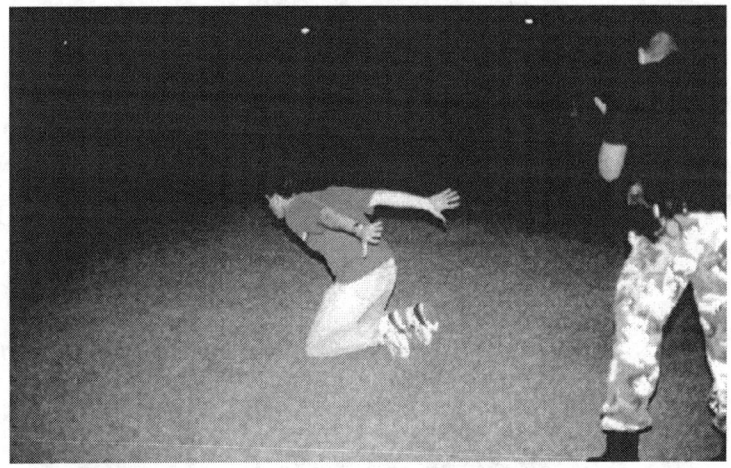

A powerful strategy in determining where to focus is to discriminate between controllable and uncontrollable factors, placing your focus on those elements you can control.

Follow the K.I.S.S. Principle

Keep it simple, warrior. Keep your concentration strategy simple, too. It is simple to get caught up trying to attend to everything that relates to training and the real world. Warriors of all walks of life have a multitude of things they are trying to manage in both training and real world situations. However, it is unrealistic to try to focus on them all.

- **Attending to too many external cues**

  Being in an intense training environment, just like a real world engagement, can be a very overwhelming experience. So many things all happening simultaneously, so many people and so many distractions. Warriors some-times get too caught up in external stimuli and forget about their internal cues.

- **Over analysis of body mechanics**

  Attending to your techniques and how you feel when executing them is important. However, sometimes too much focus on these aspects can lead to deterioration in performance. Finding the right balance of techniques focus is important in order to maintain optimal concentration levels.

A general rule of thumb is that it is realistic to attend to no more than 2-3 things during either training or operational situations. Before a mission or an intense training session, identify the 2-3 most critical things to do.

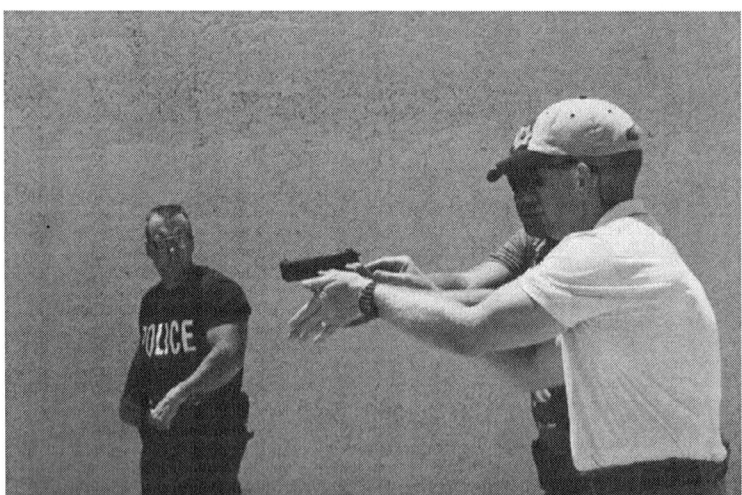

Resist the urge to overanalyze body mechanics or techniques, remember it's realistic to focus on no more than 2 - 3 things during either training or operational situations.

Dimensions of Attentional Style
(Adapted to force application training from Nideffer & Sharpe, 1978)

Now that we know a little bit about the importance of identifying where to focus your attention, the following information on attentional style may help place it in context. The following is a model developed by sports psychologist Bob Nideffer, which illustrates the four different ways warriors have found to focus their attention. Understanding the four different types of attention, and learning about your own strengths and weaknesses, are the first steps toward developing your own concentration skills. The basis for Nideffer's model is based on two theoretical assumptions. The first is that attention involves two dimensions. These dimensions are attentional width and direction. Width is the range of cues that receive attention while direction refers to the source of those cues.

Note that there are two dimensions of attention, width (on a continuum from broad to narrow), and direction (from internal to external).

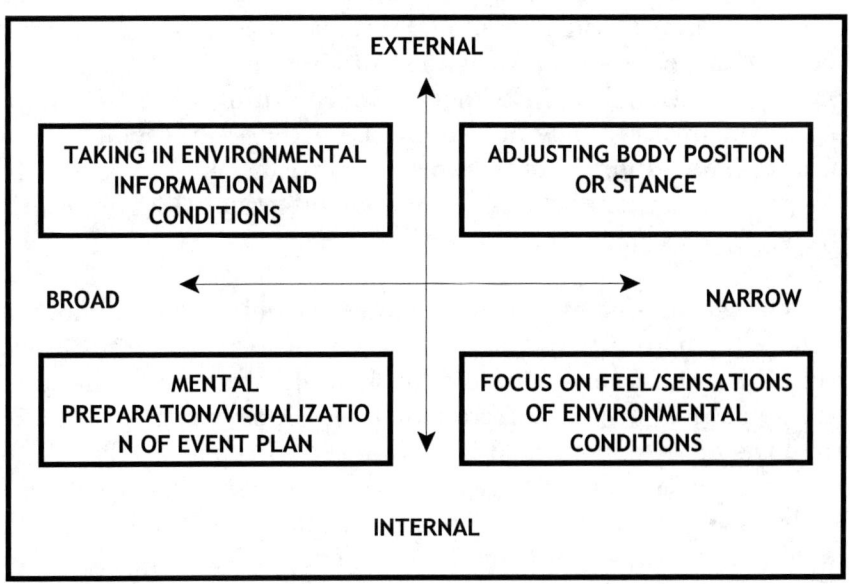

1. **Width (broad—narrow)**

   Refers to how many things you are paying attention to at once. When your attention is broad, you are paying attention to many things. When you have narrow attentional focus, you are usually concentrating on specifically one or a very few things. A football quarterback, scanning the field for receivers, has to have a broad attention, while a golfer getting ready to putt is likely to have a more narrow focus of attention.

2. **Direction (internal—external)**

   Direction is defined by whether your attention is focused internally toward your own thoughts and feelings, or externally toward the events in your environment. A marathon runner, imaging his upcoming race in his head, has an internal focus, while a baseball player up at bat, has an external focus as he watches the pitch.

The attentional requirements of conflict situations fall within the four attentional styles. For example, taking a surgical shot in compressed time frames requires a narrow-external form of attention at the moment of execution. Selecting the most effective strategy against an angry riotous crowd requires a broad-internal focus. Thus, effective attention results from adopting the appropriate attentional style to match task requirements. Flexible attention involves moving among the attentional styles as the situation demands. In other words, a warrior needs to be able to adopt all attentional styles to function effectively and appropriately.

The second assumption of Nideffer's model is that individuals tend to have attentional strengths and limitations; after all, we are all human. Some warriors are heavily analytical and don't take enough information from their environment. Other warriors read the environment well, but aren't sufficiently analytical to respond constructively. In real-world events, warriors tend to use their strongest or most confident attentional style. The weaker attentional areas often get ignored even when the situation demands it.

Individuals tend to use a broad internal focus of concentration to problem-solve, to make important decisions, to develop goals, and to anticipate the actions of an opponent under critical periods. This type of concentration requires the individual to mentally transition borders, absorb current information and use it to form assumptions about the future. When organizing inform-ation and mentally rehearsing, the same individual shifts to a narrow internal focus. At critical points in time when a detailed maneuver is required, we need to use an extremely narrow external focus and frankly speaking, we typically do. Remember basic human response under high levels of stress and the involuntary properties of the sympathetic nervous system activation. The problem is not that we don't shift to a very narrow external focus; it's that we often shift without the benefit of having a developed method of maintaining focus. Enter the overwhelming and potentially fatal effects of the human mind under stress.

To be effective, warriors must be able to shift their focus of concentration in response to the changing demands of the situation at hand. At an elite level, within an actual operational environment, success depends heavily on the internal focus, rather, to remain focused almost exclusively on the situation. When the warrior is able to do this, he or she enters a state or condition known as "the zone." When this occurs, the warrior experiences the following: (1) A perception of time being slowed; (2) A sense of complete control, and; (3) Effortless performance, with nearly automatic responses.

These experiences can be understood if you imagine the brain is a high speed camera that can snap 40 pictures every second. Under normal conditions, the brain takes an equal number of pictures in each of the four areas of concentration. Now, imagine a fight between a warrior and a dedicated opponent. The bad guy throws a punch that will take one second of travel time before it connects with the warrior's face. The warrior's perception of how fast the punch is traveling will depend on the number of pictures the brain takes of the punch. If, under normal conditions, the brain's camera is focused internally on the warrior's thoughts and concerns for half the time, then twenty pictures will be taken of the punch. With twice as many pictures to look at, the fist will seem to come at the warrior in slow motion.

Emotional Arousal

A warrior's ability to shift concentration along the dimensions of width is directly related to his or her level of emotional arousal. The higher the level the narrower the focus of concentration and the less capable the warrior is of broadening it. Whether a higher level of arousal and a narrower focus of concentration is good or bad depends on the performance demands of the environment of operation. If the warrior needs a broad focus of attention and must make adjustments to changing conditions, then a high level of emotional arousal is quite likely to interfere.

Requirements for Performance

In most situations, warriors can perform at optimal levels only when they have developed their skills to the point that those skills become automatic or reflexive, occurring void of any and all conscious direction. So long as the warrior has to mentally talk himself through his performance, or through the execution of a specific technique, this warrior cannot enter the zone. The same thing is true for a warrior who must engage in conscious thought to respond to the unexpected.

In high stress, high performance demand events, coordination and timing are all dependent on the movement of the body around its center of mass. If we draw a vertical line through the middle of the body and then draw a horizontal line, where those two lines intersect is the center of mass. Think of a kick boxer in a ring who is throwing volleys of kicks and punches with his opponent. From the onset of the bout until the final bell, there are a tremendous number of shifts in the distribution of the fighter's weight around his center of mass.

Timing allows the warrior to transfer his weight at the correct moment and it is dependent on focus of concentration and the ability to see visual indicators of cues of the impending action. It is also dependent on constant observation of the initial and subsequent actions so that speed and position can be accurately judged by the brain (speed and position of the bad guy). Any shifts of the brain's camera to internal thoughts or feelings will reduce the number of pictures taken. For that reason, adjustments the warrior makes to his stance, speed and movement, when he transfers his weight around his center of mass, must be automatic.

How to Put this Information to Use

To make use of the information in this model you have to determine which of the four attentional styles are your strengths and which styles you need to develop further. Everyone has his or her own strengths and weaknesses; some warriors are extremely good at one dimension and weak on others, while some warriors can be skilled in all dimensions.

Most frequently, elite warriors in closed skill activities tend to use a very narrow internal attentional focus. Closed skill activities include activities such as classroom training or range qualifications, because they don't have to react to changing environments or situations. For the most part their only challenge is themselves and they are more or less in control of the situations. Because classroom or range environments are typically static atmospheres, they need to be more aware of their body and overall energy management, therefore closed skill participants tend to have a more narrow internal attentional focus.

In contrast to attentional styles of warriors engaged in open skilled activities, such as driving, conflict management, and force application where the environment is fluid and constantly changing, causing the warrior to continually evaluate and re-evaluate the situation and respond. Warriors engaged in open skill activities, assuming they are properly trained, tend to use broad-external attentional skills more often than those involved in close skill activities. The other two attentional styles are important to both open and closed skill participants.

Now, through understanding the different types of attentional styles and the differences between open and closed skill activities, it's time to assess an individual's event, or the potential event they will be engaged in. Since the basis for my writing this tome is to benefit those warriors who are engaged in critical skills, we are going to assume that the event is going to be of that nature. Which of Nideffer's attentional skills is top priority in terms of the event demands and the individual's strengths? The exercises preceding this chapter are designed to help an individual or a trainer systematically review situations and determine the needed attentional dimensions.

Strategies to Enhance Concentration Skills

The following is a list of strategies and exercises that can be utilized to cultivate concentration skills.

Understanding "Where You Are" in Training

A challenge in effective concentration is figuring out the relevant things to attend to. The training environment is a perfect place to develop that understanding. In the training environment work on becoming aware of where your focus is directed. Write down where your attention is focused in a training log. After your self-awareness time, evaluate the information to identify where you tend to focus in training.

Chances are, at times your attention, or the attention of your warriors, is everywhere. The critical question to ask is how this affects performance. At times, it is okay to think random thoughts or to daydream. But, there are times when doing so will hurt performance, ultimately hurting you or others around you. At these times, where should focus be? What strategies can be used to heighten levels of concentration?

Be Realistic

Effective concentration is mentally draining. It takes energy to keep thoughts focused in relevant, controllable, beneficial directions. It is not necessary or very realistic to expect oneself to focus throughout training or an operational situation. However, it is important to identify the critical moments when one needs to attend to the task at hand. It is these moments when an individual wants to kick in focus.

Use Cue Words

Cue words are a form of self-talk (see chapter five). They are designed to trigger a specific response, either instructional or motivational. For example, you can use cue words to direct attention back to task. If the mind begins to wander, using cue words such as "focus" can help you remain on task. Likewise, motivational cue words serve to remind you of the task at hand. If you feel yourself paying too much attention to the wrong thing when you're executing a warrant in a hostile neighborhood, saying "mission" to yourself can bring you back to the task at hand.

Practice with Distractions Present or Making the Training World Real

So often training sessions are calm, predictable and controlled, not anything like the real world. Trainers, it may be beneficial to set up training times with varying distractions present, such as sighs, sounds and smells like those found in the real world. By exposing warriors to typical real world distractions they can be somewhat inoculated to their effects and they can learn to focus past them.

Practice Shifting Attention

We have identified four general quadrants of attention and acknowledged that the situation, in part, dictates the appropriate attentional focus. Given this, a critical skill is the ability to shift—to go from a broad external to narrow internal focus. The training environment is the optimum place to experiment with shifting attention. Choose multiple places to direct your attention (i.e. stances, target, breathing, movement, opponent). Then set intervals through the various attentional directions. Practice shifting. It will make the skills easier to use in an operational format.

Routines

Creating and practicing operational skills in a routine can help focus your attention and concentration on the right things at the right time. An operational routine is a set of actions that you take each time before a planned real world event. The routine could include a warm up, imagery, and visualization.

Controlling Distractions

Once a warrior is capable of performing and making adjustments without having to consciously think about it, we are ready to begin working on learning to control distractions or those thoughts and feelings that interfere with performance in actual, real-world events.

In most real-world conflicts, it is not the warrior who has the perfect performance who wins; instead it is the warrior who makes the fewest mistakes, and/or the warrior who recovers from minor problems quickly. Because we know that mistakes will be made, and that unexpected events will take place in conflict (remember: predictably unpredictable), it becomes critical that warriors have some strategies or techniques to reduce the amount of time it takes them to let go of distractions and refocus concentration to meet the challenge. To briefly describe what happens to concentration, physiology, and performance in a critical event, when a warrior loses his edge, we will start with a highly confident warrior.

The loss of an edge sends a pattern of stimuli to the brain that says something is wrong. That pattern is perceived as a threat and causes almost instantaneous changes in the warrior's body. Physically, muscles tighten and breathing and heart rate accelerates. The focus of concentration narrows; instinctively and automatically the warrior begins to make changes in body position in an attempt to recover balance and normality in the situation.

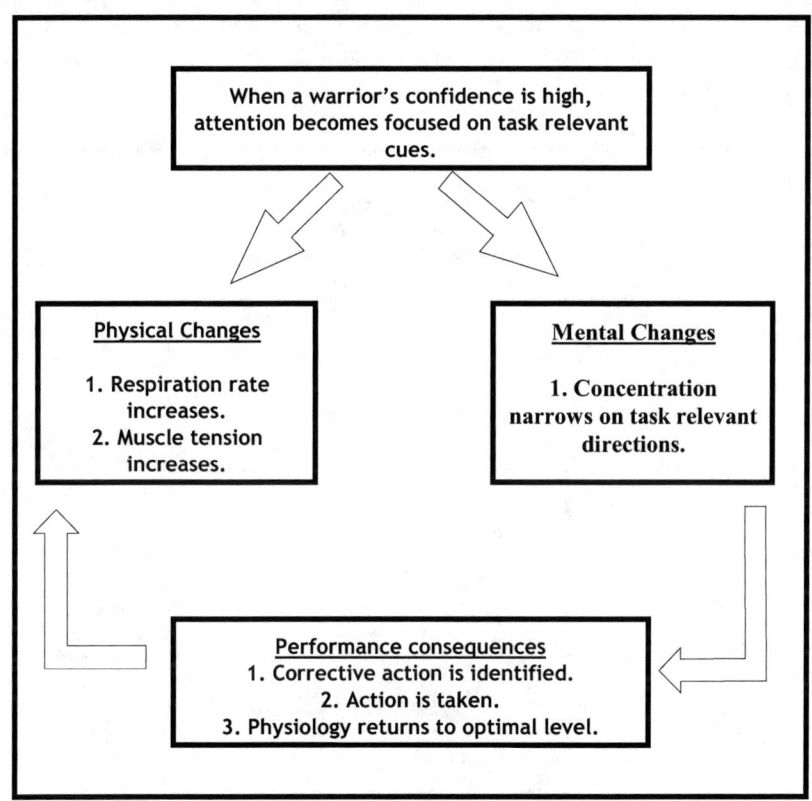

The confident warrior becomes aware very early in the recovery process that he is regaining control and will not have much of a problem recovering. His confidence allows him to let go of any thoughts and concerns and to almost immediately relax and get back to work. For the confident warrior, the loss of an edge and the adjustments that had to be made required little in the way of conscious internal processing. As a result, the warrior was able to maintain external focus. His perception of time wasn't sped up that much and he didn't lose any awareness of the situation; perceptual time loss was minimal.

When a warrior lacks confidence, the recovery processes are slowed and this can have an extremely dramatic effect on performance. The longer muscles remain tense, the longer it takes the warrior to get back into the fight. The warrior loses time, and without flexibility in his body the likelihood of problems increases. Focus on concentration remains narrow and the warrior fails to see cues that allow him to anticipate his opponent and set up properly for techniques. If he fails, the anxiety and concern that contributed to his situation will increase as does the likelihood of greater problems.

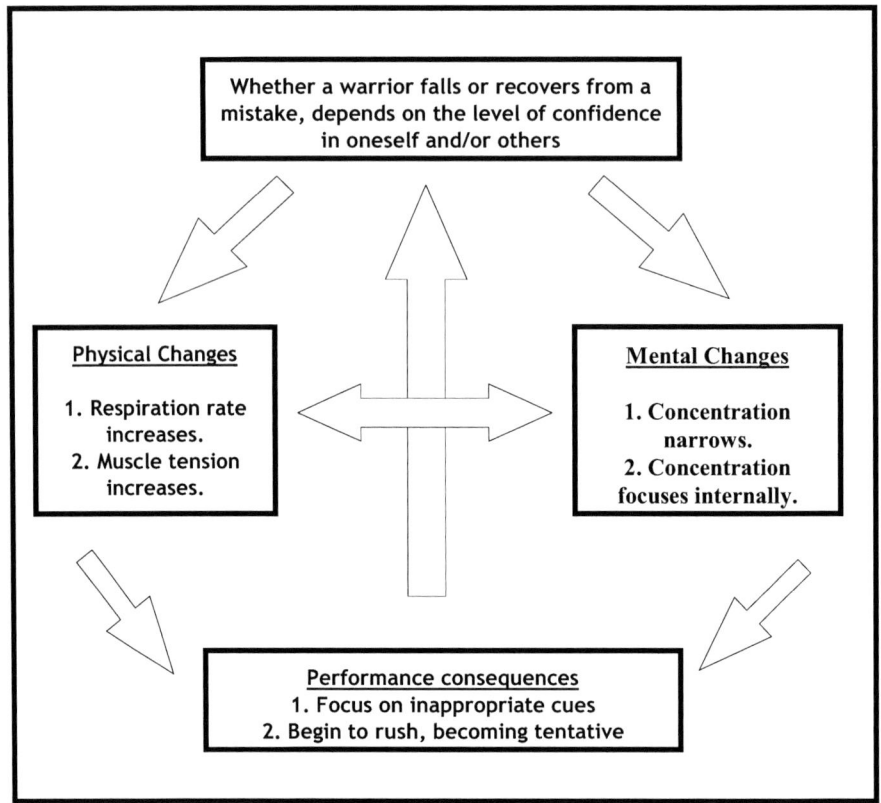

Centering

To assist warriors in recovering more quickly, we need to teach them to use a simple breathing technique to help them regain control over both physiological changes that have occurred and their focus of concentration.

Warriors should be taught to use the length of time it takes to exhale, to consciously attend to their level of muscle tension, especially in their shoulders and lower body, and to quickly adjust those tension levels and their body position relative to their center of mass, so that they feel "centered." This occurs when the pattern of stimulation the brain is getting from the warrior's position signals everything is okay. That momentary conscious internal monitoring of feelings shouldn't take more than a second of the warrior's time. In that second, however, the warrior has let go of distractions and has completed his or her recovery. The warrior is back in position, ready to rock and roll!

Center of mass, Centered & Centering

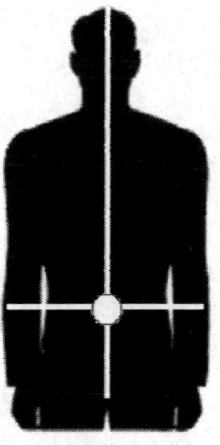

- o **Center of mass is a physiological spot located in the center of the body.**

- o **Centered is a feeling you have when you are confident and ready to perform.**

- o **Centering is the process you go through to achieve a feeling of being "centered."**

> # TRAINER'S GUIDE

So how do you teach concentration? How can you tell a warrior to think and concentrate? How do you know that he or she is actually improving concentration skills?

We know from experience that there will be an infinite number of distractions in a real-world situation. If the warrior isn't totally confident, and most of them are not, then these distractions can become the difference between winning and losing, life and death. As part of our perception, we want to minimize possible distractions, by anticipating as many as possible and being able to adjust appropriately. This is where solid experiential style training comes into play. For example, in the time immediately following the Columbine High School shooting, agencies became concerned with the possibility of an active shooter situation in their jurisdiction. Training to combat these incidents were held in schools and office buildings around the nation, all with relative surprisingly positive results. However, most of the initial training programs only addressed the mechanics of moving and clearing and failed to address the potential distracters present in active shooter events. When the training events were modified and included such things as: active fire alarms, screams, running and interfering victims, injured, IED's, and active fire suppression systems, the results were very different and not nearly as favorable.

Get Their Attention...

Older and More Experienced Warriors

At the end of this chapter is a concentration grid. It is an easy method to demonstrate the power of concentration to your warriors. The grid is 10 x 10 with numbers from 00 to 99. This is a timed task; typically trainers allow about 1 minute for each time through the grid. Begin with the sheets turned over. Have the students break off into pairs—one does the exercise while the other acts as a distracter. Explain to each of the students that they are supposed to start with 00. Put an X in that box when they find it and then move on to 01, 02, 03, etc. The distracter tries to divert the attention of their partner by talking or yelling at them. At the end of the minute have your students tally the number of boxes they have checked off. Before discussing the exercise, have them switch roles.

When you have finished working with the grid exercises ask some follow-up questions: How did your partner impact your performance? At your best, how were you focused? What happened when you got distracted? Then make the application to the training environment. Discuss how distractions impact performance and emphasize the need for effective concentration.

Younger and Less Experienced Warriors

Prepare a small field with 10 to 20 different items on it such as: a pistol, a magazine, a knife, a baton, a book, etc. Give your warriors 1 minute to study the items and during this time play some sort of distracting music and play it loud. At the end of the minute, instruct the warriors to write down as many things as they can remember. Follow up with questions similar to the first exercise.

Training Concentration

- Ask your warriors to define concentration and have them explain why it is important.
- Talk about controlling the controllables. Ask your warriors to list things they can and can't control in both training and in the real world. Use this as a lead-in to figuring out where to direct attention.
- Depending on the ages of the warriors in your charge, present the four attentional styles and have your warriors identify their strengths and their weaknesses.
- Cover some of the common concentration problems along with skills to help prevent these problems.
- Use some of the exercises to help warriors become aware of their own concentration practices.

Exercises to Develop Concentration Skills

Several exercises have been included to help you hone your concentration skills, or those of the warriors in your charge. The following is a brief description of these exercises.

Exercise 1a and 1b can be used with both older, more seasoned warriors and younger, less experienced warriors. It asks the warriors to determine where their attention is focused in many different situations. Once attentional style is determined the warriors can then work to improve their concentration.

Exercise 2 includes several ways to practice focusing under high pressure, high stress situations. These exercises are designed for the more seasoned warriors, but may be modified for newer individuals if need be.

Exercise 3, 3a and 3b are included to help warriors establish a refocusing routine. Exercise 3 takes the warriors through creating a refocusing routine. Exercise 3a and 3b can be used as supplementary refocusing sheets, adding some more structure to the way warriors refocus and plan for the inevitable lapses in concentration.

Finally at the end of the chapter a concentration grid is included to use in the "Get their attention…" exercise.

CONCENTRATION - Exercise 1a
Identifying Concentration Tendencies

After intense training, do your best to recall how you were focused—what you were attending to in the following situations. After completing the third session, go back and assess how the focus impacted your performance (positive, neutral, or negative). In cases where the impact was neutral or negative, identify how you would prefer to focus in those situations.

DAY OR SESSION 1

BEFORE TRAINING:

DURING DRILLS:

DURING CLASSROOM PERIOD:

FOLLOWING TRAINING:

DAY OR SESSION 2

BEFORE TRAINING:

DURING DRILLS:

DURING CLASSROOM PERIOD:

FOLLOWING TRAINING:

DAY OR SESSION 3

BEFORE TRAINING:

DURING DRILLS:

DURING CLASSROOM PERIOD:

FOLLOWING TRAINING:

CONCENTRATION - Exercise 1b
Where am I focusing?

Use this exercise to help identify your tendencies related to attentional style.

DURING HIGH REPETITION DRILLS:

DURING STATIC RANGE DRILLS:

DURING DT DRILLS:

WHEN DISCIPLINED:

WHEN RECEIVING PRAISE:

WHEN EQUIPMENT FAILS:

WHEN HAVING A BAD DAY:

WHEN HAVING A GREAT DAY:

WHICH ATTENTIONAL STYLE(S) DO MOST OF YOUR ANSWERS FIT INTO? WHICH ATTENTIONAL STYLE(S) DO YOU NEED TO WORK ON?

CONCENTRATION - Exercise 2
Focus under pressure

In the following are several ideas for ways to practice focusing under pressure.

1. Change of Focus Drill

Select a period of time (from 30 seconds to 2 minutes) during which you direct focus to only one aspect of a drill, skill, or technique. Change focus during the following time interval.

For example, you might switch your focus among the following areas:

- Movement – how is my stride?
- Turns and pivots – how is my body position?
- Breathing – am I breathing easily?

How else might you practice switching your focus?

2. Simulation Training

Re-create a real-world or challenging training event in practice. Simulated experiences enable you to become much more familiar with event-specific stimuli, to the point where that stimulus no longer represents a distraction.

3. Distraction Drills

Practice executing drills or mission-specific skills despite verbal, visual and environmental distractions. For example, during a range exercise, have roll players or teammates yell distracting comments or verbally taunt the warrior, Overhead lights, sirens, smoke, are also possible distractions and ones that could be encountered in the real-world. During the exercise allow your mind to switch back and forth between wandering and bringing your thoughts and focus back.

4. Quality Practice

This exercise design is brief and intense. You must be ready as soon as training begins. You have only one opportunity to execute a specific drill, for a specific time frame and/or distance. Over time, your ability to focus intensely while performing well will increase.

CONCENTRATION - Exercise 3
Building a refocus routine

1. *Recognize Distractions*

   Identify the factors in training and the real-world which are likely to distract your attention or draw your focus away from crucial elements of performance.

2. *Select Your Focus*

   Identify the factors in your performance, which require your concentration. Where should your focus be?

3. *Prepare to Concentrate*

   Concentration requires a passive, relaxed mind. It is helpful to begin to recognize and reduce stress and anxiety. Too much stress destroys attentional focus. While it may be unrealistic to keep your environment stress-free, pay attention to the stress you can control or limit versus that which is out of control and therefore not worth focusing on.

4. *Create Concentration Cues*

   Use attentional words, images, or actions as reminders to concentrate. Called "cues," these words, images, or actions should be simple, positive and personally meaningful.

5. *Create Your Own Refocusing Routines*

   Anticipate possible distracters and decide how you will respond to them. These responses are your refocusing routines. Practice these until they are effective and instinctive. If you plan what you will do between events or training days, you will find you can bring your concentration under control. Refocusing routines reduce uncertainty and decrease susceptibility to distractions.

   During your training periods, make a mental note of the distractions that interfere with your concentration. Record this information in the graph on the next page. Do this immediately after training or during a break while the experience is still fresh in the memory.

CONCENTRATION - Exercise 3
Refocus form A

DISTRACTIONS	COPING RESPONSE TO MINIMIZE NEGATIVE IMPACT	ATTENTIONAL CUE
EXAMPLE: NEGATIVE THOUGHTS AND SELF-DOUBT.	EXAMPLE: IMMEDIATE THOUGHT STOPPING TECHNIQUE, POSITIVE AFFIRMATION.	EXAMPLE: VISUALIZE STOPPING.

CONCENTRATION - Exercise 3
Refocus form B

Use the situations provided below or supply your own as you anticipate and plan for the unexpected (Orlick, 1986).

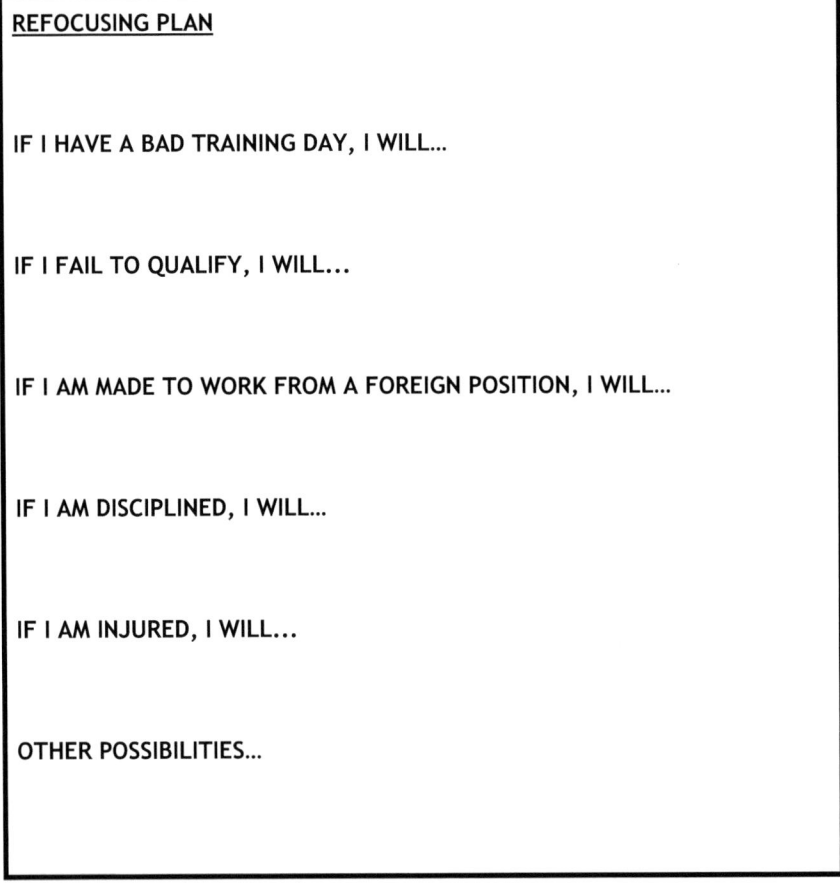

REFOCUSING PLAN

IF I HAVE A BAD TRAINING DAY, I WILL...

IF I FAIL TO QUALIFY, I WILL...

IF I AM MADE TO WORK FROM A FOREIGN POSITION, I WILL...

IF I AM DISCIPLINED, I WILL...

IF I AM INJURED, I WILL...

OTHER POSSIBILITIES...

38	28	51	09	71	16	72	82	63	04
10	32	44	62	21	97	18	40	90	52
25	85	57	46	66	35	78	96	11	69
74	03	75	93	00	56	22	67	49	20
43	13	23	33	79	95	76	05	59	45
65	86	50	19	41	07	37	83	29	61
58	02	34	77	27	55	92	48	01	89
15	47	73	87	39	68	12	53	84	70
24	64	81	06	91	60	88	30	98	14
99	31	42	94	17	54	80	26	36	08

Chapter Eight

TEAM BUILDING: TRAIN THE INDIVIDUAL AND TRAIN THE TEAM

"The achievements of an organization are the results of the combined effort of each individual."

— Vince Lombardi

Why Team Building in What Is Often an Individual Pursuit?

Take a pencil and a piece of paper, write a list of why you like your job or ask your warriors to list why they like their jobs.

Your list will likely look something like the following:

1. It's fun
2. It's exciting
3. It's rewarding
4. I like working with my team/squad mates
5. I want to be a better person or help others
6. It's a great way to serve my community/country

Somewhere on most warriors' lists is something to the effect of "I like working with my teammates or squad mates." When performance-based psychologists study reasons for participation, usually one of the top reasons is social interaction, like: "to be with friends," "co-workers." Although spontaneous conflict is often an individual pursuit, the warrior and the bad guy(s), interactions in training and in real world events with peers helps to shape the overall experience. A positive environment with trainer, supervisors, administration and warriors all supporting each other can lead to tremendous individual success.

This chapter will focus on several aspects of teamwork. First, we'll look at how a group becomes a team, the process that takes place and how to assess where a team is in this process. Second, we will discuss specific characteristics of highly successful teams. In doing so, for each characteristic, we will provide a description

171

and explanation of the characteristic, an example related to conflict management, and strategies for trainers developing these characteristics in their teams. Finally, we will provide exercises to be used to facilitate individual warriors becoming a team.

How Do Individuals Become a Team?

Group development generally follows a specific process. The most common model for explaining how individuals form as a group was developed by Tuckman (1965). This model suggests that when developing into a group, individuals go through four distinct stages:

- Forming   • Storming   • Norming   • Performing

While the progression from one stage to another may be perceived as linear, in many cases teams can waiver back and forth between stages before actually progressing on to the next stage. Let's look at each of these stages and apply them to warrior development.

• Forming

During the forming stage, the potential team members usually come together for the first time. This is a learning period for old and new members, acquainting and re-acquainting themselves with how the group functions, their roles within the group and the goals of the group. In order to facilitate this stage, trainers or supervisors often set up time outside of training for social activities such as a get-together, BBQ, or party to allow the group to get to know each other better. This is also the time when trainers or supervisors go over the rules of the group, be they formal or informal.

• Storming

The storming phase usually occurs a short period into team development, depending on the amount of training time allotted. This may be within a few weeks or even as late as a month. The honeymoon period is over at this point and it's time to get to work. This phase is characterized by conflict over who has control and infighting for status positions and the trainer's or supervisor's attention. It is during the storming phase that those warriors with poor work ethic, and/or bad attitude, emerge; personality and goal conflict among team members also become apparent. While it seems like a counterproductive stage, keep in mind that the storming phase is inevitable and if channeled correctly can lead to effective team building. Trainers and supervisor's need to be vigilant in identifying conflicts when they emerge and open up communication paths to resolve the conflict in a timely manner. Successful resolution can lead to increases in team member's self-esteem, respect for their teammates' similarities and differences, overall trust and communication skill effectiveness.

- **Norming**

The calm after the storm. Norming is the period after the storming where the team has come to a consensus about what is acceptable and what is not. Goals, objectives and expectations have been clearly defined by the trainer and by the warriors. The respect they gain for their teammates unique contribution to the team is the most important realization the warriors come to during the norming phase.

- **Performing**

The performing stage is similar to the peak at the end of the training cycle. During this stage, there is a close bond among group members and a general want for one another to succeed. The team members begin to truly value each individual's contribution and the relationships are secure within the team. The group is finally acting as a confident cohesive unit. In this final stage, the team should be able to combine effort towards the group goals.

Having an awareness of the four-stage process of becoming a team can be helpful in a couple of ways. First, it provides a structure to what has probably been witnessed in the training or operational environment. Observed behaviors and relationships can now be placed into a defined context. Second, by understanding each of the stages, proactive steps can be taken to facilitate the successful progression through each of the stages, to promote successful team formation and growth.

Characteristics of Successful Teams

To enhance trainer effectiveness, one strategy used is to identify characteristics of successful trainers and try to develop these characteristics in other trainers. We can take a similar approach when trying to understand and enhance team effectiveness. First, we need to identify the characteristics of successful teams. While teams are successful for a multitude of reasons, six characteristics deserve special attention. Specifically, successful teams usually have **clear goals**, a high degree of **commitment** from team members, **clear roles** for each team member, a high degree of **respect** for each other, pathways for **open communication** and **consistent training/supervision**. Each of these six factors will be discussed in detail. After each description, exercises will be provided to be used to develop the given characteristic in high-performance teams. Note that many of these traits that make teams successful can be developed as a team progresses through the four stages of forming a team.

- **Clear goals**

The first characteristic of successful teams is clear goals. Effective goal setting for individual warriors was discussed in detail in chapter three of this book. It may be beneficial to review that chapter because when setting team goals many of the same principles still apply—be specific, use long-term and short-term goals, set task and outcome goals and be flexible and realistic. However, setting team goals is sometimes more challenging because the whole team has to agree on where they are going and how they are going to get there. The goal setting process is often facilitated by asking the team at the beginning of the training cycle, **"What can you as a group achieve?"** This process gets the team thinking about the realm of possibilities as well as their motivation and commitment to the goal.

End of the Career Party

Exercises to facilitate team goal setting is to have your team split up into small groups and ask them to identify how they would like to be remembered at an end of the career or retirement party. Ask each group to report to the other groups how they think the team should be remembered at the end of a career, what legacy do they want to leave behind? This exercise will serve as a way to start discussions about the group goal (where they want to be) and team mission.

Mission Statement

Once the group has brainstormed about where they want to be at the end of the road, have them formalize their goals into a mission statement. A mission statement is a way to clarify team dreams into team goals. Remember that for the goal to be effective it must be specific; ideally, the mission statement will give purpose and direction to the training cycle and the year at hand. Once created, the team should post the mission statement either in the training area or some sort of common area as a daily reminder of where they want to go.

• Commitment

Involving the team in the creation of the team goals and mission process is the first step to gaining their commitment as it leads to increased motivation as well as feelings of ownership and accountability. If the warriors are not involved and don't feel like their input is valued it is very likely they won't feel a level of commitment. Commitment is best viewed on a continuum with commitment level fluctuating throughout the training period and throughout the team building process. It is when commitment is at the extremes that one should be concerned. In the book, *Championship Team Building*, Jeff Janssen (1999) defined eight stages of commitment. Can you see these in yourself or your teammates?

- **Resistant**—Someone who has not bought into the team goal; they are working on their own agenda and are usually very selfish.

- **Reluctant**—This person is hesitant, disinterested and afraid to commit to the team goal, and typically do just enough to get by.
- **Existent**—To this person the team goal has little significance; they are just working because all their peers are.
- **Complaint**—The team goal is important to this warrior. However, they do just enough to get by, no more and no less.
- **Committed**—This type of warrior views the team goal as very important. They will do anything they can to achieve it, such as putting in extra time and energy.
- **Compelled**—To this warrior, the team goal is of utmost importance. They are totally invested in it and it becomes their true mission. These warriors thoroughly enjoy the extra time they put in.
- **Apathetic**—Someone who doesn't care and has lost all love for the work.
- **Obsessed**—To this person, the goal is the only focus; they partake in extreme behaviors such as overtraining.

A successful team is made up of a balance of compliant, committed and compelled individuals. Given this, a challenge for trainers and supervisors is to identify the commitment levels on your team and strategies to effectively train and develop each type of warrior and possibly influence their commitment level.

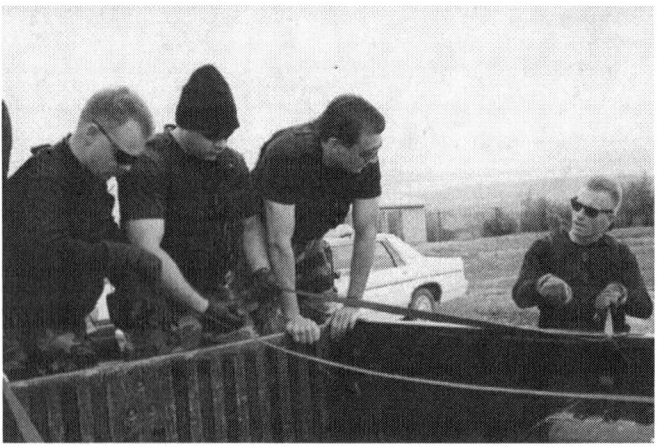

Winning teams are a balance of complaint, committed and compelled warriors.

Influencing Commitment

It is often the less committed warriors that are the most challenging (those further down the continuum than compliant). In order to reach these individuals, challenge them to make the commitment by emphasizing their responsibility to the team. It is often productive to have each warrior tell the group what he or she is going to do to help the team achieve its goal. Another strategy is to have a one-on-one talk with them to understand why they aren't making the commitment (or is afraid to make the commitment).

Team Practice

During regular training, assign several of your warriors to design training. By doing so, you are in essence saying that their input counts. Often when the individuals are allowed to design and execute their training they are very likely to work harder because they truly enjoy the session they have developed for themselves.

Specific Roles

In each and every team, team members take on certain constructive roles whether it be team leader, counselor, social director, motivator, or class clown.

- **Team Leader**—The warrior, who through his/her actions, both physically and emotionally, sets the tone for the team.
- **Counselor**—The warrior who helps struggling or troubled team members and often acts as peacemaker in times of dissension.
- **Social Director**—The warrior who is always planning ways to get together outside of work so the team can bond.
- **Motivators**—Highly spirited warriors who can get the team up with their behavior and language.
- **Class Clowns**—These warriors lend some of their sense of humor to the training and the operational environments, tend to help make training and real world call-ups much more enjoyable events.

The key to becoming a successful team is getting each member to accept their role as well as see value in the other roles both in and out of team activities.

- **Understanding roles**

This exercise is designed to help your warriors understand each other's roles. All you need is a ball. Have your team sit in a circle facing each other. The first warrior takes the ball and tosses it to a teammate (anywhere in the circle). The warrior who threw the ball then talks about the things the team needs from the teammate who caught the ball in order for the team to be successful. The warrior with the ball then repeats the process by tossing the ball to another teammate and talking about the things the team needs from that teammate in order to be successful.

After each team member has been talked about and has had a chance to speak, begin a discussion about what the exercise means to the team. More than likely they will talk about how each member of the team is dependent on the other. To further the discussion, get them to think about what would happen if one member of the team were no longer around.

- **Respect**

It is important for a team to understand and accept that not everyone is going to be best friends. While friendship among team members isn't a critical element of successful teams, respect is. When talking to your team about respect, remind them that they can earn respect of their teammates through the actions and attitudes they display daily in and out of team activities.

Identify Noteworthy Behaviors

In every training session, ask one of your teammates to select a teammate who has consistently demonstrated exemplary behavior in training and at work. Ask the individual to give a specific example of something this warrior did and how it impacted the team. Such an exercise can illuminate positive behaviors and facilitate mutual respect.

- **Open communication**

Communication comes in many different forms and at many different levels. Trainer-warrior and warrior-warrior communication should be open. That is, trainers and warriors are encouraged to honestly express themselves about team standards, individual and team goal, feelings, and expectations. Remember to keep an open door policy when communicating with your warriors as well as to check in with your warriors from time to time to see how they are doing and feeling. Encourage your warriors to communicate both compliments and complaints.

Effective communication involves both the sending and receiving of messages. Let's review a few basic criteria to keep in mind when communicating. The following are several guidelines when sending messages (Janssen, 1999).

- **Be direct**—Speak directly to the person you would like to talk to.
- **Be complete and specific**
- **Be consistent**
- **Communicate your needs and feelings**
- **Be concise and focused**

In high-performance pursuits, an important aspect of sending messages relates to giving feedback. Janssen (1999) sets out six guidelines for giving feedback.

1. **Be positive**—Your warriors will respond better to the feedback if it is stated in a positive manner.
2. **Be specific**—Let your warriors know what he or she did well or exactly what he or she needs to improve.
3. **Give the feedback immediately after the performance**—Doing this will reinforce the good behavior and help to change the undesirable behavior.
4. **Be sincere and honest.**
5. **Give feedback less often when skills are learned**—This tends to build confidence in your warriors.

6. **Focus on effort as well as results**—Not everyone on the team can be number one, so structure feedback so that it reflects each individual's performance, not their performance as related to other team members.

In addition, when correcting mistakes as part of feedback, use the "sandwich technique"—meaning try to sandwich the critique between two positive comments. Start by relaying a positive comment, follow that by a correction (what they should do) and end with encouragement and hope.

As mentioned, effective communication involves two components: sending and receiving information. Receiving information requires the skill of listening. You may be the best communicator on your team, however if your team members are not listening this will get you nowhere. Listening shows that you care about what your teammates and team members are saying, and what they are saying is important to building a successful team.

• **Consistent training and supervision**

Trainers and supervisors serve an important role in bringing the team together. Often, without the guidance and support of the trainer, the team doesn't have a chance at being successful. There are three major factors that make up consistent training and supervision:

Fairness, Dedicated Staff, and Consistency

Fairness

In order to promote cohesiveness, commitment and satisfaction within a team, the trainer/supervisor needs to demonstrate fairness in his/her leadership style and decisions. Fairness can be demonstrated by

• Making a conscious effort to ensure that the trainer's perceptions of the warriors are not having a negative impact on interactions with the warriors.

- Being aware of attention and interest that is paid to different individuals. Find positive things each team member is doing and help each member improve their skills.

- Keeping lines of communication open. This will aid in the perception of fairness on the team and in the organization.

Dedicated Staff

Know your stuff!!! Being a trainer and a leader takes up a lot of time, but most people are in the profession because they love it! Continue to show your warriors your dedication in the way you walk, talk, and act. They will be more likely to buy into what you are saying if they understand your commitment to them.

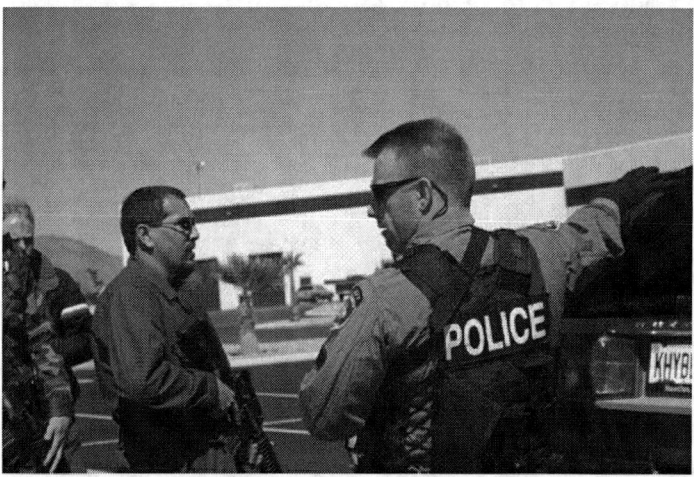

For cohesiveness and commitment in a team, the leader needs to show unquestionable fairness in both leadership style and decisions.

Consistency

Trainers and leaders who change their minds at the drop of a hat do not gain the respect needed to create a cohesive team. They end up confusing their team instead of leading their team to great accomplishments. Trainers who have repeated success are consistent in their philosophies and standards. I am not suggesting that you should never make improvements to your philosophy or standards; however, the most successful teams know what their leaders expect of them in every training session, on every mission.

How to Use This Information

To begin incorporating these characteristics into your team, the first step is to assess the current status of your team. You may find that they already possess some of these characteristics. Next, identify the characteristics that would be beneficial to try to instill within your program. Prioritize—don't try to do it all now. Then, develop a plan. How will respect be bred amongst warriors and leaders? Or, how can you monitor the fairness displayed by the leadership staff? As with anything that is of value, it doesn't come easily. Hard work and commitment to change is critical.

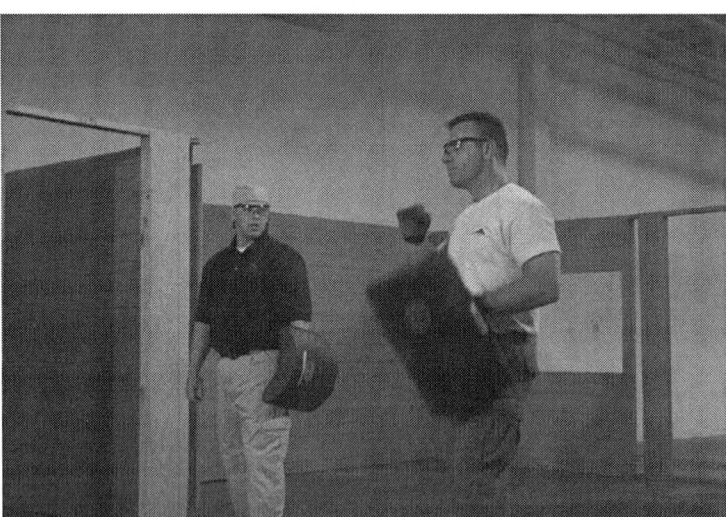

Anything of value doesn't come easily. Hard work and commitment to change is critical.

Chapter Nine

PHYSICAL AND MENTAL ENERGY

"Victory is the beautiful, bright-colored flower. Transport is the stem without which it could never have blossomed."
— Winston Churchill

Managing Energy to Facilitate Performance

At the most basic level, you can't perform at a high level without enough energy, just as you can't drive a car without gas, watch TV without electricity, or listen to iPods without batteries. Warriors must have good stores of energy and use them wisely. Success, in part, is based on the proper control of a warrior's energy level. Too low, and you may not have the intensity you need to battle a tough situation or opponent. Too high, and you may be too wired or nervous to perform a complicated skill. "Optimal" energy level is very individualized which means that two individuals on the same team, with the same training and similar backgrounds, may perform best at very different energy levels.

Read through the following two examples that illustrate how energy levels can impact performance.

1. Dave is in a five-man stack getting ready to breach the front door of a home on a felony warrant service detail. This is his first time at such an event. He is so nervous he is shaking and feels like he is going to vomit; his muscles feel tight and all he can think about is not screwing up. How do you think he is going to perform?

2. Bob is excited, almost anxious, to get through the door on the same warrant service. He knows he is ready to cover his areas of responsibility on this entry; he is prepared for the challenge, and knows he needs to focus on the mission at hand. How do you think Bob will perform?

Energy management can be the difference between making it through the event safely and ending in tragedy.

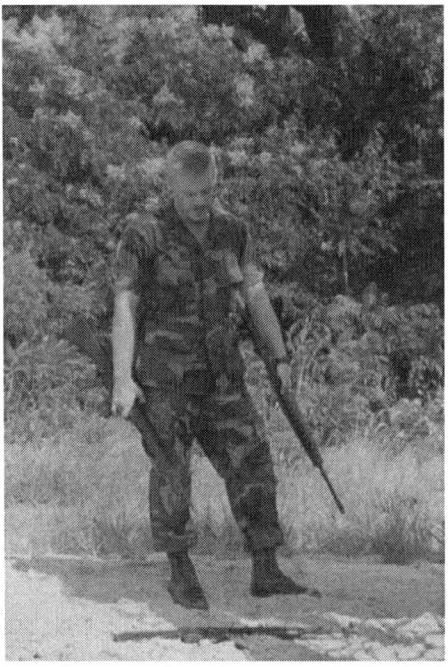

Warriors need to have good physical and mental energy. Success, in part, is based on the proper control of a warrior's energy levels.

Understanding Energy

A first step in learning how to manage energy is to recognize the two types of energy—physical energy and mental energy. Physical energy relates to the activation level of your body from low energy (lethargic) to high energy (heart racing, jittery). Mental energy relates to the activation level of your mind from low (no motivation) to high (racing thoughts, excessively worried). This distinction is critical because different strategies will be used to target mental versus physical symptoms. In both training and real world events, you have an energy level (physical and mental) at which you perform well. The challenge is to manage your physical and mental energy levels so they can help your performance in both training and in the real world.

What Affects Your Energy Level?

It is sometimes useful to think of yourself as a battery in that you can either be "zapped" of physical and mental energy or you can be "charged" with physical and mental energy. Other people, events, and things can affect your physical and mental energy; knowing how things affect your energy can help you and your warriors better manage it. Complete the table below to help identify what zaps you and what charges you.

	Examples	You
Zappers	Poor Sleep Poor Eating Negative people Worry/Stress	
Charges	Motivational music Confidence Physical skill Memories	

Strategies to Manage Energy Levels

Now that you are aware of what zaps and charges you, let's take it a step further and discuss specific strategies you can use to manage your physical and mental energy. In doing so, we'll also discuss symptoms related to too much or too little energy to help you identify when you need to put these strategies into play. One of the strategies, deep or diaphragm breathing, will be discussed in detail at the end of the chapter as it is useful when trying to manage excessive nervousness—an all too common ailment of elite warriors.

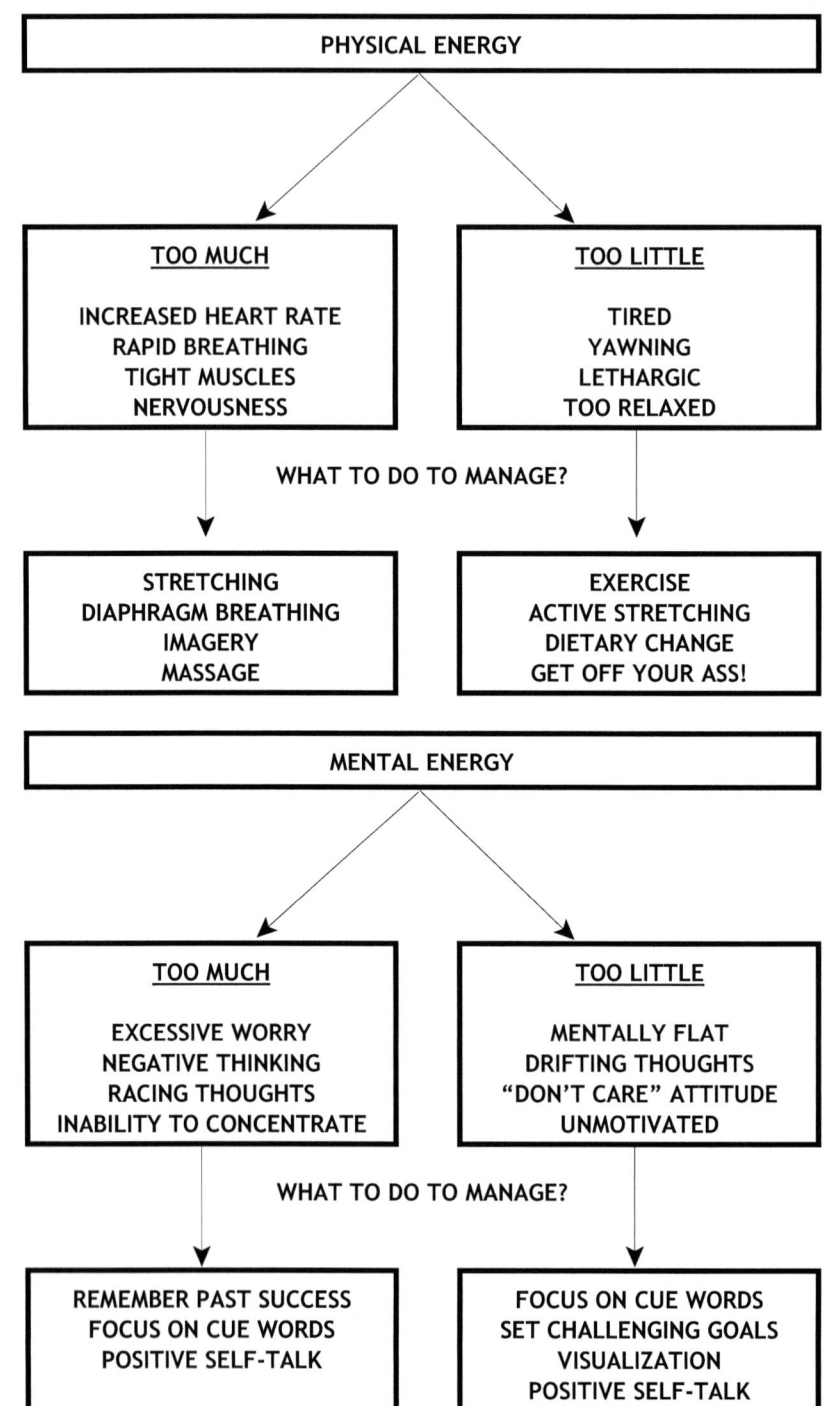

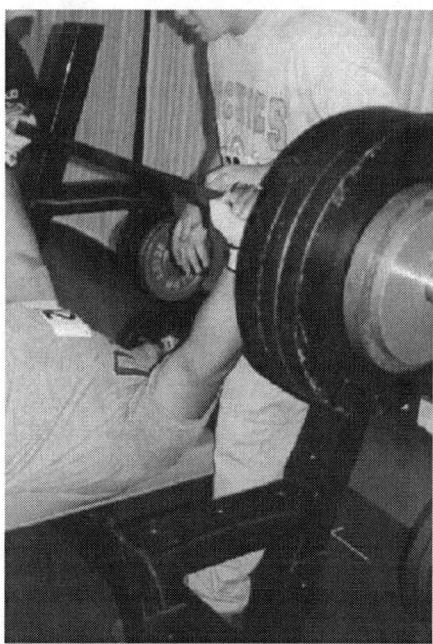

The importance of managing energy in training and real world events cannot be over-emphasized. Developing strategies to help you and your warriors manage energy levels needs to be part of your training program.

Now that you know about physical and mental energy, the importance of managing energy in training and real world events, and strategies to help you and your warriors manage energy levels...It is time to GET STARTED! Begin with monitoring your mental and physical energy levels in training. Use some of the strategies outlined in the previous figures and finish at the end of the chapter when you feel your energy is either too high or too low. Then, once you have practiced these skills and strategies, use them in the real world to help manage energy.

$$\boxed{\text{TRAINER'S GUIDE}}$$

- Begin by describing what is meant by energy level.
- Talk about the two types of energy levels: mental and physical.
- Read the descriptions of the two types of warriors and have your warriors guess which one is going to perform well and which one isn't.
- Remind your warriors that not everyone is the same; what might be right for one is totally wrong for another.
- Have your warriors fill out the chart that identifies both their drains and charges.
- Talk about these charges and drains and help your warriors develop strategies to get them in the right energy zone.
- Take some time to teach your warriors diaphragm breathing. Some warriors may need to use this technique to calm down before every actual operation, whereas others may only need to use this skill occasionally.

Exercises to Develop Mental and Physical Energy and Manage It

The following exercises are designed to help you become aware of your energy levels and control them in both training and in real-world events.

Exercise 1 can be used in conjunction with the earlier section on zappers, to help warriors recognize what charges them and zaps them.

Exercise 2 can be used to help warriors of all ages and all skill levels to understand what energizes them and what depletes their energy levels.

Exercise 3 takes warriors through a series of questions helping them to discover their optimum energy level for performance.

Exercise 4 teaches warriors a relaxation method to help them control their energy levels when they are too high.

ENERGY - Exercise 1
What are your charges and drains?

	EXAMPLES	YOU
DRAINS	POOR SLEEP NOT EATING RIGHT NEGATIVE PEOPLE WORRY STRESS	
CHARGES	MOTIVATING MUSIC BEING CONFIDENT BEING PHYSICALLY FIT BEING PREPARED	

ENERGY - Exercise 2
What affects your energy level?

WRITE DOWN 3 THINGS THAT CHARGE YOUR PHYSICAL AND MENTAL ENERGY IN TRAINING	WRITE DOWN 3 THINGS THAT ZAP YOUR PHYSICAL AND MENTAL ENERGY IN TRAINING
1.	1.
2.	2.
3.	3.
WRITE DOWN 3 THINGS THAT CHARGE YOUR PHYSICAL AND MENTAL ENERGY IN THE REAL-WORLD.	WRITE DOWN 3 THINGS THAT ZAP YOUR PHYSICAL AND MENTAL ENERGY IN THE REAL-WORLD.
1.	1.
2.	2.
3.	3.

How much control do you have over these charges and drains? One step in increasing your energy for training and real-world events is to take charge of your environment, adding as many charges as you can, and eliminating as many drains as you can. Make an energy plan for real-world operational events, and then make one for training sessions.

ENERGY - Exercise 3
Find the right energy level

To operate well, it is critical for warriors to know what energy level works best for them. We know, from research and experience with elite athletes and military special operations personnel, that warriors can be physically and mentally over-activated, leading to nervousness, muscle tension, and/or attention problems. We have also seen warriors who simply can't get fired up enough to mentally focus or activate their bodies for the challenges at hand. To figure out the ideal energy level for you, think of your 3 best and 3 worst performances. Try your best to remember how you felt before and during those events.

BEST	LOW		MODERATE		HIGH	
MUSCLE TENSION	1	2	3	4	5	6	7
HEART RATE	1	2	3	4	5	6	7
BREATHING	1	2	3	4	5	6	7
DOUBT/WORRY	1	2	3	4	5	6	7
NEGATIVE THOUGHTS	1	2	3	4	5	6	7

WORST	LOW		MODERATE		HIGH	
MUSCLE TENSION	1	2	3	4	5	6	7
HEART RATE	1	2	3	4	5	6	7
BREATHING	1	2	3	4	5	6	7
DOUBT/WORRY	1	2	3	4	5	6	7
NEGATIVE THOUGHTS	1	2	3	4	5	6	7

I assume there is a difference between your best and worst performances in terms of what was going on related to your physical and mental energy. How do you think your physical and mental energy levels influenced your performance? What can you do to create this physical and mental energy level prior to events?

ENERGY - Exercise 4
Gain control / relaxation

We all know how to breathe, we do it every day without knowing it, and it doesn't even take practice. However, if controlled properly, we can use breathing as a form of relaxation during high stress and critical times.

Controlled Breathing

Breathing is one of the easiest physiological systems to control. If done correctly, breathing can have a calming effect on the body by delivering the appropriate amount of oxygen to the body as well as working to remove waste products associated with physical labor.

Breathing from the Diaphragm

Diaphragmatic breathing is a key component to using the breath as a relaxation tool. To learn diaphragmatic breathing follow these steps.

1. Lay down on your back. Place one hand by your side and the other on your abdomen, on top or just below the navel.
2. As you breathe, concentrate on using your diaphragm to fill your lungs. You will know when you have done this by the way your abdominal area expands each time you take a breath. The hand you placed on your abdomen should rise and fall each time you take a breath. Try not to raise your shoulders as you breathe in.

Rhythmic Breathing

Rhythmic breathing involves breathing to a measured count. For instance you might inhale for a count of four, hold your breath for a count of four and exhale for a count of four. While doing rhythmic breathing become aware of each breath you take. Try to fill your lungs completely when inhaling, as well as completely exhaling by squeezing your muscles to eliminate all the air. Also pay attention to the period of time when you are holding your breath. Become aware of the tension felt in the muscles as well as the releases of this tension when you are exhaling.

Ratio Breathing

Ratio breathing consists of using a specific ratio for breathing. For instance a 2:1 pattern, When using this ratio you might breathe in for a count of four and exhale for a count of eight. At first you may have to concentrate heavily on the breathing pattern. However, as you become better at controlling your breathing, these breaths should become automatic.

Learning to control your breathing over time will help to improve overall balance, power, and coordination, which eventually will lead to a greater tolerance for the physical discomfort associated with training and injury.

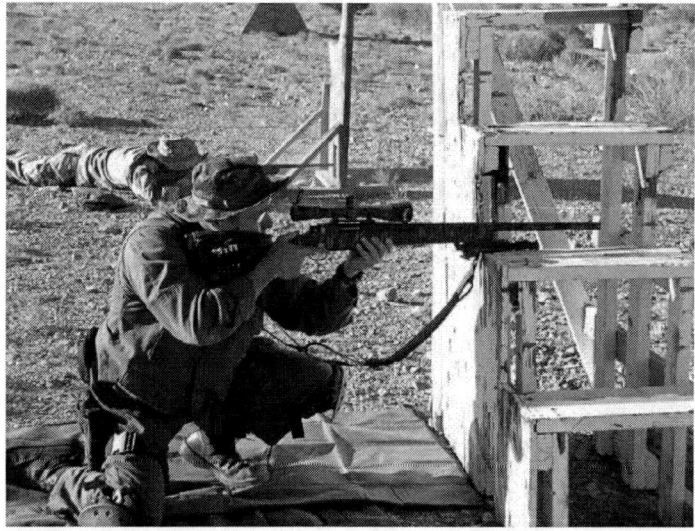

Control techniques, like those used by precision marksmen, help to improve balance, power, and coordination, leading to a greater tolerance for the physical discomfort associated with training and injury.

Chapter Ten

PUTTING THE MENTAL WITH THE MECHANICAL: PUTTING IT ALL TOGETHER

"Man is only truly great when he acts from his passions."
— Benjamin Disraeli

As odd as this sounds, real world events provide warriors with opportunities. The opportunity to demonstrate their abilities; to challenge themselves as to how efficiently they can respond under the real pressures of the world. To do things for real is one of the reasons that warriors train hard on a regular basis. When stacked at a door waiting for the knock, it all boils down to what one's body can do, right? **WRONG!!** Let me provide you some examples to illustrate why performance is much more than physical capabilities and mechanical skills.

Example A: John spent half an hour prepping his gear and getting suited up. He is now adjusting his goggles waiting for the go-ahead to load up in the deployment vehicle. He has reminded himself of his hard work in training so his confidence is high. His focus is on exploding through the mission, maintaining a consistent tempo, and holding his areas of responsibilities. He is set to be the number 1 man in the stack, but he doesn't care because all he is thinking about is **HIS** performance and what he needs to succeed.

Example B: Robert spent the last half an hour prepping his gear and getting suited up. He is now adjusting his goggles waiting for the go-ahead to load up in the deployment vehicle. He has trained hard all year, but questions whether he did enough to prepare himself. He is set to be the number 1 man in the stack, but is worried about performing well because he feels the need to have visual contact with his teammates. He is so anxious about performing that he can't seem to remember **HOW** to do his part of the mission.

In comparing John and Robert, it seems that both are physically prepared for operational work. They have trained hard and have readied their bodies to perform. Are both going to perform well? OH, HELL, NO! While John is both physically and mentally prepared to perform, Robert has not taken control of his mental preparation. To put it another way...When a warrior steps up to the plate to perform, both his or her body and mind are with them. Because of this, warriors better make sure both their body and their mind are prepared to perform. In this chapter, we'll discuss steps warriors can take to ensure their mind is working for them and not against them in real world endeavors.

"Nothing can stop the man with the right mental attitude
from achieving his goal; nothing on earth can help
the man with the wrong mental attitude."
Thomas Jefferson, 3rd President of the United States

The discussion and examples above should convince warriors of the importance of operational mental preparations (OMP). But, for those who are still not sold on the value of mental preparation, read on as some research findings related to characteristics of elite athletes and warriors are described:

- Just like scientists have identified physical, physiological or technical profiles of elite athletes, similar work has been done related to identifying psychological profiles of elite performers. Their results have identified numerous psychological skills and characteristics related to success. These include **having a well-developed, competitive or operational routine,** high levels of motivation and commitment, coping skills, self-confidence and arousal management.
- After the 1996 Olympics, researchers tried to identify the factors that had a positive and negative impact on performance during the events. One of the findings that distinguished those athletes that performed well from those who did not was the **development and adherence to physical and mental preparation plans.** Successful athletes had a pre-competition routine that they stuck to!

- In 1998, ten athletes from the U.S. were interviewed, to uncover how they approached/dealt with the mental aspect of competition. In particular, each athlete was asked to describe how he/she got ready to win. Interestingly, even though the athletes prepared for their events differently, **all of the athletes had a routine or plan to get mentally ready to win.**

Interesting support, isn't it? Mental preparation seems to be a critical factor related to success. While some individuals "sort of" have a way to get them in the mood to perform, the preparation routine tends to be used consistently. Just like the other psychological skills in this manual, your mental preparation, in concert with physical preparation, must be developed systematically and purposefully, practiced, refined and used consistently in order for it to be effective.

Understanding Mental Preparation Routines

To prepare physically to perform, most individuals have some sort of standardized training regime they go through. Some have individualized this training to include routines that optimally prepare the body for the rigors of arduous work, like running, weight training, etc. They do what they feel is best for them and not necessarily what their teammates are doing. A similar approach should be taken regarding mental preparation in that a warrior should have specific thoughts, words, images and feelings leading up to a real event, to optimally prepare the mind for expeditious and appropriate response. This mental routine often occurs in conjunction with physical and mechanical preparation as the warrior is training his body and his mind.

Benefits of Developing and Using a Mental Preparation Routine

Now that everyone is convinced of the importance of mental preparation, it is probably critical to identify the benefits of developing and consistently using a mental preparation routine. Doing so will enhance commitment when warriors are asked to change their behavior or to dedicate time to mental preparation. Some benefits include:

Attain an Ideal State or "Zone"

The primary benefit or purpose of a mental preparation plan is to get the warrior in a "mental state" that seems to relate to success performance (for the individual).

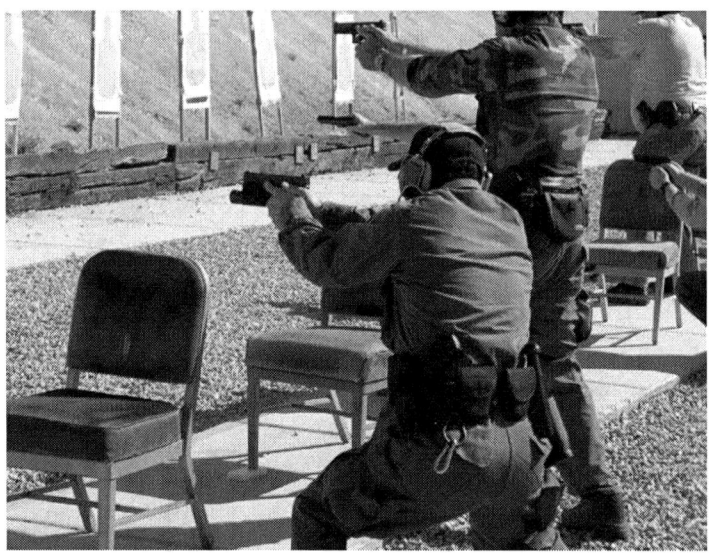

When warriors step up to the plate to perform, they must ensure both their body and their mind are prepared to achieve.

High Self-confidence

Success breeds confidence! When a warrior is able to see and feel past and future successes as part of his/her mental preparation, confidence is not far behind. Imaging a successful upcoming event is the "dress rehearsal" to the real deal. Visualizing a great performance enhances the warrior's belief that they can truly do it!

Control of Mental Energy

As discussed in an earlier chapter, it is critical to manage mental energy so the individual is not too flat or too manic. During preparation, warriors can listen to motivational, driving type music, to get wound-up about a pending event or imagine a peaceful and relaxing scene to slow their thoughts down. Such strategies can be a purposeful part of mental routine to manage mental energy.

Effective Focus

A mental preparation routine can help the warrior focus on important aspects of performance. Technical cues ("You can do it," "fight!") or images ("tank," "explode") can be integrated into preparation to direct attention where it needs to be (as opposed to having one's focus on unproductive or negative things).

Comfort in Structure

A mental routine can be a security blanket—something to turn to in a stressful moment leading up to an actual event. It is a mental routine they can use whether they are performing a traffic stop or clearing a cave in Afghanistan; to bring consistency to their preparation and to their performance. To a degree, a mental preparation routine can help take the environment out of the performance (for those who tend to be negatively affected by environmental conditions).

Engage the Mind

The mind is a valuable tool. When purposefully recruited and engaged, the athlete has the additional support of positive emotions, feelings and thoughts. Warriors should make wise use of all resources at their disposal.

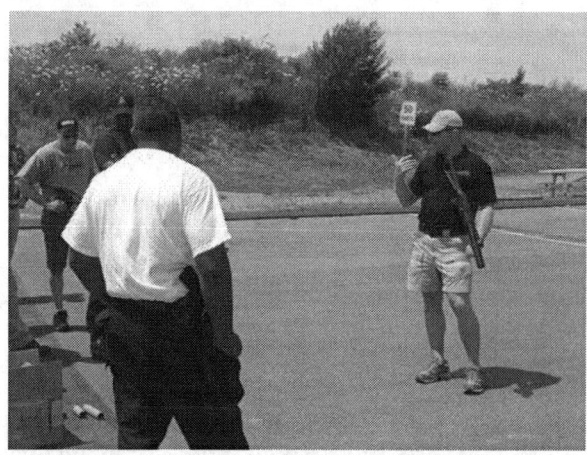

The mind is an indispensable apparatus. When recruited and engaged, the warrior can gain support from positive thoughts and emotions.

Putting the Pieces Together

Now is the time to put all the pieces together. It's like a puzzle. We have supplied all the mental tools that the warrior needs to excel. Choose the tools wisely and put them together in the form of a mental preparation plan. Two steps need to be taken by warriors to complete the puzzle:

First, the athlete needs to figure out the desired results. Which is, how does the warrior want to think and feel, in training and in a real world event? What mindset seems to relate to successful operations for a warrior? Does he or she want to be very confident, nervous, relaxed, happy, a little worried, controlled, high energy, etc? At the end of the chapter are exercises that can help individuals determine the mindset that may be best for them.

Second, the warrior needs to determine how he or she is going to get into this mental state. What tools are they going to use to attain the ideal mindset? Following is an example to bring this to life. As part of an interview, a world championship team athlete was asked to describe in detail how he prepares himself for competition. He discussed specific things he does, thinks, and says to himself prior to the event. Then, he noted that "I need to be nervous before I compete" (awareness of an ideal state/desired end result of preparation). Great! The next question, of course, was how do you get nervous? "Simple, I stare at my competitors in the ready room" (this is part of the process he uses to attain his desired state). He also identified other mental tools he uses to get himself mentally ready for competition.

Following are some mental tools that may be useful in helping warriors to attain their desired mindset:

Goals

While outcome is certainly important, the immediate focus and goal should be directed toward what the warrior needs to do. Remember, effective goals can help motivate and direct attention. Make sure the goal is directing and motivating appropriately.

Self-talk

Before the event, internal talk should be positive, motivating and instructive. Cue words can be included that tell the warrior what to do to perform well and help build confidence.

Mental Imagery

Imagery is often used to rehearse the event and event strategy to prepare the warrior for the challenge ahead. It can also be used to take the warrior away from the stressful environment.

Performance Cues/Concentration

Eyes and ears should be directed to the task ahead. Concentration strategies can be used to ensure an appropriate focus.

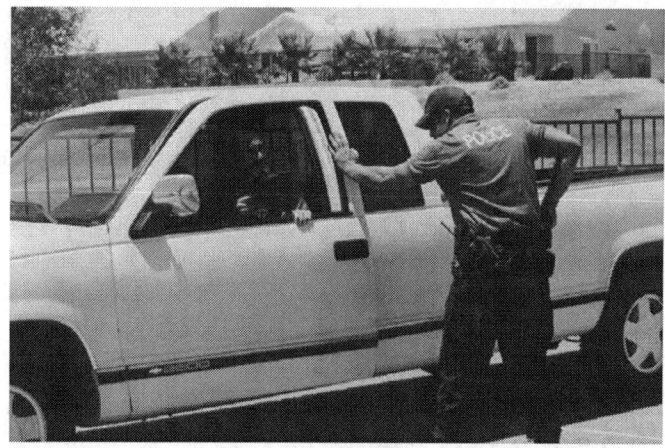

The senses need to be directed to the task at hand. Concentration strategies are designed to ensure an appropriate focus.

Relaxation and Activation

It is critical for the warrior to manage physical and mental energy. Warriors should have at their disposal a variety of strategies to attain an effective energy level.

┌─────────────────────────────────┐
│ TRAINER'S GUIDE │
└─────────────────────────────────┘

- Start by talking to your warriors about what mental preparation is and why it is important to have a mental plan.
- Define some of the key components that make up a mental plan, such as imagery, goal setting, self-talk, concentration, and energy management.
- Explain to your warriors that there is no right or wrong way to create a mental plan. Each warrior will have his/her own personal mental plan.
- Have your warriors take some time to complete the reflections exercise. Explain to them the importance of being honest on this exercise.
- Next have your warriors examine their reflections exercise and begin to understand how they feel when they perform well and what they need to do in order to ensure good performances. Also, make sure they examine how they feel when they do not perform as well and what they need to do to get out of this state.
- Now have your warriors spend some time creating a mental plan.
- Set up a training day and during it let your warriors practice their mental plans. Give them a chance to do their own mental preparation. This will allow them to take ownership for their readiness routine and allow them to make changes if needed.

┌───┐
│ **EMPHASIZE THE IMPORTANCE** │
│ **OF WRITING ALL THIS DOWN!** │
└───┘

Mental Preparation Exercises

Exercises 1 - 3 are designed to help warriors think about how they feel in their best and worst conditions. Exercise 1 is adopted from the competitive reflections form, developed by Orlick (1986). Its main purpose is to get older, more seasoned warriors thinking about how they feel and act when they are performing well and how they feel and act when they are not performing well. Exercise 2 and 3 are similar forms developed for newer, less-experienced warriors. From these forms each warrior can begin to create their own individual mental plan.

Exercises 4 and 5 are similar worksheets designed to help warriors of all skill levels in creating mental and physical plans. Exercise 4 is for newer warriors while Exercise 5 is for more experienced warriors.

MENTAL PREPARATION - Exercise 1
Real-world reflections

How do I get started on developing a routine that will work for me? Begin with the end in mind. You need to identify how you need to think and feel to perform your very best. Then, you need to identify what to do to get you into this ideal mindset. It is helpful to refer to past experiences to figure out what seems to work for you. Respond to the questions from this form (Orlick, 1986) to help you get started on developing a mental routine that will work for you.

Think of your best performance in the past year and respond to the following:

1. *How did you feel just before the event?*

NO ACTIVATION											HIGH ACTIVATION
											MENTALLY/PHYSICALLY
MENTALLY/ PHYSICALLY FLAT	1	2	3	4	5	6	7	8	9	10	CHARGED
NOT WORRIED/ SCARED	1	2	3	4	5	6	7	8	9	10	EXTREMELY WORRIED

2. *What were you saying or thinking to yourself before the event began?*

3. *How were you focused during the event? What were you aware of or paying attention to during the event?*

Now, consider your worst performance in the past year when responding to the following:

4. *How did you feel just before the event?*

NO ACTIVATION											HIGH ACTIVATION
MENTALLY/ PHYSICALLY FLAT	1	2	3	4	5	6	7	8	9	10	MENTALLY/PHYSICALLY CHARGED
NOT WORRIED/ SCARED	1	2	3	4	5	6	7	8	9	10	EXTREMELY WORRIED

5. *What were you saying or thinking before the event began?*

6. *How were you focused during the event? What were you aware of or paying attention to during the event?*

7. *What were the major differences in your energy level and your thoughts prior to these two situations? What was your focus of attention during each event?*

Review your responses to the questions from the reflections form. In particular, note the differences between your thoughts, focus, and energy level before your best versus your worst performance. How would you prefer to think or feel before you perform? How would you prefer to focus before and during the event? With this in mind, you now need to begin figuring out specific strategies to help you reach this optimal mindset. For example, if you tend to perform your best when you are intense and aggressive, identify specific things you can think, say, and do to help you attain this feeling. Or if you tend to get overly anxious when you think too much about the event, figure out what you can do to purposely distract yourself until moments before the event. (Motivational music, self-talk, etc.)

8. *Before I perform, my optimal state of mind consists of:*

9. *Strategies to help me achieve my optimal state of mind include:*

MENTAL PREPARATION - Exercise 2
How do you feel/act (best)

Take some time to think about your best performance ever. Write about what you were thinking, what you were feeling and how you were acting before, during and after the event.

WHAT/HOW WERE YOU	THINKING	FEELING	ACTING
BEFORE THE EVENT...			
DURING THE EVENT...			
AFTER THE EVENT...			

MENTAL PREPARATION - Exercise 3
How do you feel/act (worst)

Take some time to think about your worst performance ever. Write what you were thinking, what you were feeling and how you were acting before, during and after the event.

WHAT/HOW WERE YOU	THINKING	FEELING	ACTING
BEFORE THE EVENT...			
DURING THE EVENT...			
AFTER THE EVENT...			

MENTAL PREPARATION - Exercise 4
Real-world event plan

Take some time to look at your worst and best performance sheets. Use the information on these sheets to create a real-world event plan. Examples of elements to possibly include in your mental preparation: mental imagery, cue words, positive self-talk, diaphragmatic breathing or other relaxation strategy and reminders about your goal. In the boxes relating to your physical readiness you could write down what you like to do to prepare and how you need to feel physically.

	WHAT YOU NEED TO DO TO BE MENTALLY READY?	WHAT YOU NEED TO DO TO BE PHYSICALLY READY?
1 HOUR BEFORE THE EVENT...		
10 MINUTES BEFORE THE EVENT...		
DURING THE EVENT...		
SPECIFIC TIME INTO THE EVENT...		
FOLLOWING THE EVENT...		

MENTAL PREPARATION - Exercise 5

Take some time to look at your worst and best performance sheets. Use the information on these sheets to create a real-world event plan. Examples of elements to possibly include in your mental preparation: mental imagery, cue words, positive self-talk, diaphragmatic breathing or other relaxation strategy and reminders about your goal. In the boxes relating to your physical readiness you could write down what you like to do to prepare and how you need to feel physically.

	WHAT YOU NEED TO DO TO BE MENTALLY READY?	WHAT YOU NEED TO DO TO BE PHYSICALLY READY?
10 MINUTES BEFORE THE EVENT...		
1 MINUTE BEFORE THE EVENT...		
DURING THE EVENT...		
CRITICAL TIME DURING THE EVENT...		
FOLLOWING THE EVENT...		

Burnout, Short-term and Long-term

Since the context of this manual is performance enhancement, both for the here and now and for years down the road, it
is only right to address the issue of burnout.

Burnout is a debilitating condition which happens as a
response to stress over a period of time. It may manifest itself
psychologically, emotionally or physically, and generally occurs
in stages of severity. The first symptoms may be fatigue,
frustration, irritability or an overall lack of motivation, and if
unchecked it may deteriorate to feelings of helplessness, lack of
control, and even physical symptoms such as headaches or
chronic back pain.

Burnout can affect anybody, but the people most susceptible
to it are those who are extremely dedicated high-achieving, and
goal oriented. Some people with these characteristics do manage
to cope effectively; resisting stress and avoiding burnout, but
more often these high-achievers refuse to accept the fact that
they have limitations or weaknesses. They are likely to blame
others, or blame circumstances beyond their control, before they
will admit that their problem came from themselves, and much
is based on their perception of themselves and their
circumstances.

Burnout in the world of the warrior usually occurs as a result
of working or training too hard, for too long with little apparent
reward. It also happens when warriors do not give themselves
enough variety in the type of training they do or the type of real-
world events they are involved in. Obviously, I am a huge
proponent of training to win and the concept of winning, hence,
the first book, and, of course, this book; and there can only be one
winner. Even if the loser in the event achieved outstanding
things the rewards of putting forth the effort to win and
ultimately being that winner is second to none. Of course, there
is no trophy in conflict, losing usually means dead or incapaci-
tated.

Warriors can avoid burnout and circumvent the long-term
effects of stress by having realistic mental training programs. It

is essential to have expectations which are in line with reality; individuals need to be careful not to judge themselves or their team by unrealistic standards. Goals should be challenging, but they should also be achievable, and it is important to create a realistic time frame by which to interpret results. Warriors who try to achieve all that they desire in a single training session or short time frame are setting a virtually impossible task for themselves. Hard work is essential, but must be kept in perspective. Warriors will find that they will benefit more if they do whatever is necessary to remain enthusiastic and excited about their occupation, they should not lose sight of the fact that they chose to do the work they do (See the difference between survival and winning in *Train to Win*), and that they chose it because they love it!

When training for the ugliness of the real world it is crucial for individuals and teams to provide variety in their training programs and to have sufficient down time between training evolutions and real-world events. The best time to take time off is when they are still enthusiastic about their job, instead of when their performance goes downhill. Burnout in the world of warriors develops fairly rapidly, especially when people who normally train or deploy occasionally, are thrust into fulltime training or fighting.

Too many warriors fail to ensure that they have sufficient time off, they take days off only when they are told to. This is me speaking from experience, I would only take leave when I transferred from duty stations and while working as a civilian cop. I didn't take vacation during the first 8 years I was on the job, this does not provide for any break in routine. If a warrior put just a little more emphasis on mental training rather than doing as much physical training as humanly possible, putting more thought into a training program which develops both psychological and physical skills, they can keep burnout at a minimum. It is sad to see warriors who have great talent and potential, but who are not achieving the results they deserve because they are neglecting the psychological skills required for peak performance.

Instructors and Trainers Get Burnout, Too...

Operational warriors are not the only ones who suffer from burnout and the long-term effects of stress; it can also be a serious problem for trainers. When teaching warriors, frequently it is easy to become burnt out; to lose energy and enthusiasm. This may lead to a dull and jaded instructor and consequently a lower rate of student interest or retention; and instructor burnout seriously contributes to a higher rate of student injuries.

For warriors and trainers suffering burnout, the immediate solution is to check their goals and re-establish their direction. They must increase their self-awareness and be honest about what is important to them. It is also essential that they accept that they are solely responsible for their own actions and behaviors—and that other people are responsible for theirs.

It is important for everyone to realize that burnout is a very normal reaction to stress; it is not a disease and cannot be cured by pills or shots. Burnout is usually a product of poor approaches to reality and training, in other words a psychologically-induced problem. Obviously, mental training can help warriors to deal with it and to ensure that they are not suffering from its complications.

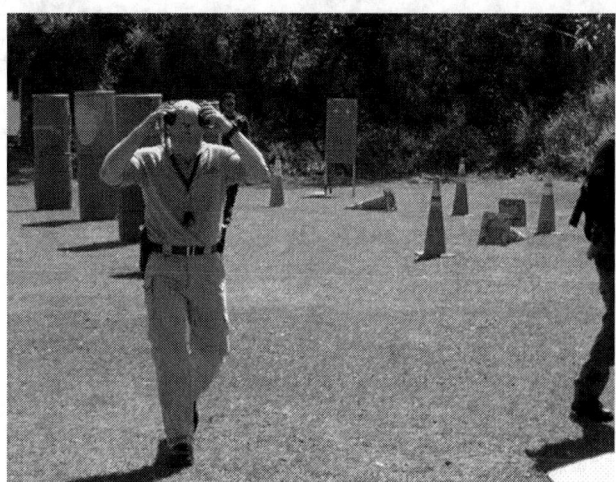

Burn out can lead to a mind-numbing and jaded instructor, consequently resulting in lower student interest, retention and even contribute to injuries.

Skills for Life

Contemporary research indicates that future success emanates totally and absolutely from a person's mental attitude and self-concept (Porter, 1986). If the warrior accepts the previously covered material, that the individual mind has real and actual power, the warrior can understand the importance of those concepts. If, in the mind, we visualize ourselves failing we can actually manifest that into a reality.

What is the mind? It is that thinking part of the organism called man—the visions, the thoughts and the dreams—the part of the individual that talks to itself, analyzing, creating, thinking. It is the part of the warrior that separates him from animals, lower in the food chain. In any case it is the part of you that is responsible for creativity, thinking and problem solving. You can change your mind through the use of powerful tools because they help you condition and recondition your thinking and reframe your experiences into positive, learning situations. This allows you to create a new, better, more productive reality with your mind and your emotions.

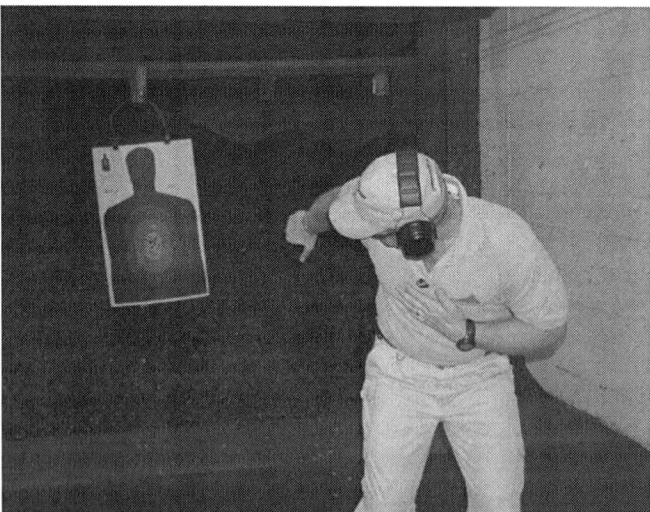

The warrior can condition and recondition individual thinking and reframe experiences into positive, learning situations. Creating a new, better, more productive reality.

Conclusion

In this guide, I have examined mental training as used by elite athletes and suggested ways in which it can be used successfully by warriors. There can be no doubt that a well-structured mental training program, when combined with quality physical and mechanical training, will produce better prepared warriors with faster skill acquisition and higher performance levels than ever before.

For warriors to achieve the performance level they are capable of, they need to make use of the mental training techniques which have proved to be of benefit in other like endeavors. Warriors have a tendency to set themselves apart from other walks of life—but in the final analysis being a modern warrior is like any other voluntary pursuit, and like any other pursuit in life, warriors cannot expect to achieve their full potential if they do not include mental preparation in their training. There is much more to becoming a great warrior than simply throwing a punch or pulling a trigger!

The majority of U.S. law enforcement officers and trainers feel that the greatest challenge facing their undertakings is a lack of administrative and financial support, which makes it difficult and expensive to gain a high level of experience and readiness. It also isolates this warrior path from new methods, techniques and equipment. Consequently, mental training would appear to be of particular value to these wonderfully dedicated folks, as it costs nothing and can simulate much of what they need to do without actually having to be there! When the number of training days and bullets are limited by a lack of finances, facilities, injuries, or administrative red tape, a good mental training program can pay dividends.

So, whether you're a warrior or a trainer of warriors, if you work on the techniques described in this book, they will help you to improve the warrior you want to be. You can make things much easier for yourself. Mental training works—if you choose to use it.

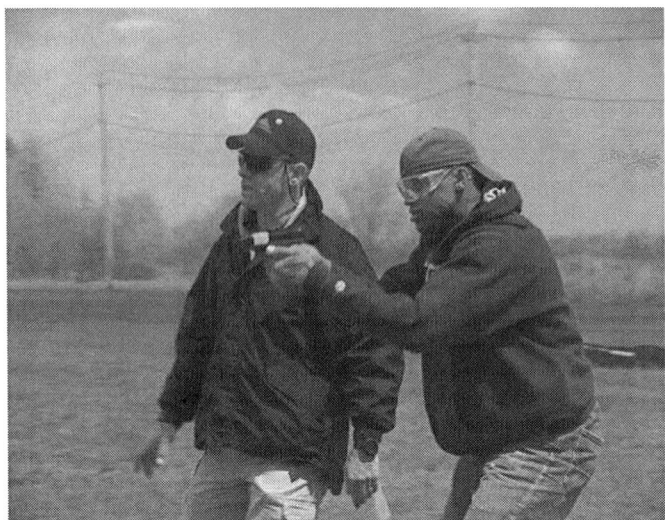

For warriors to achieve the performance levels they are capable of, it is important to make use of mental training techniques, proven to be of benefit in other high demand activities.

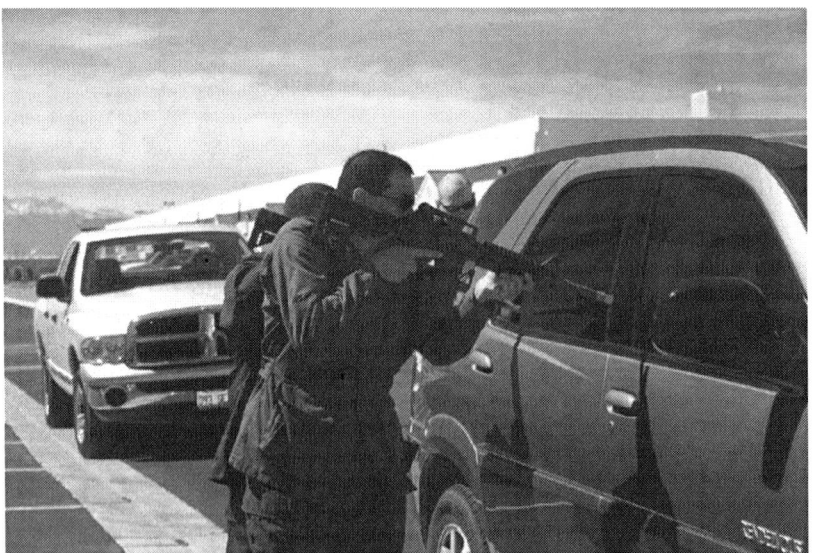

Warriors tend to set themselves apart from others—but being a warrior is like any other thing in life, warriors cannot achieve full potential without mental skills, after all there is much more to being a warrior than simply throwing a punch or pulling a trigger!

YOU ARE WHAT YOU THINK YOU ARE

If you think you're beaten, you are.
If you think you dare not, you don't
If you'd like to win, but think you can't
It's almost certain you won't

If you think you'll lose, you've lost
For out in the world we find,
success begins with a person's will
It's all in the state of mind

If you think you're outclassed, you are
You've got to think high to rise
You've got to be sure of yourself
Before you can ever win a prize.

Life's battles don't always go
To the stronger or faster man
But sooner or later the man who wins
Is the man who thinks he can

Author
Anonymous

REFERENCES

Adams, J.A. (1961). The second facet for forgetting: a review of warm-up decrement. Psychological Bulletin, 58, 257-273

Adam, J. J., & van Wieringen, P. C. (1988). Worry and emotionality: Its influence on the performance of a throwing task. International Journal of Sport Psychology, 19, 211-225.

Anderson, J.R. (1980). Cognitive psychology and its implications. New York: W.H. Freeman

Annett, J. (1995). Motor imagery: perception of action? Neuropsychologia, 33 (11) 1395-1417

Baron, R.A., Byrne, D., & Watson, G. (2005). Exploring social psychology (4th Canadian edition). Toronto, Canada: Pearson.

Behm, D.G. & Sale, D.G. (1993). Intended rather than actual movement velocity determines velocity-specific training response. Journal of Applied Physiology, 74 (1), 359-368

Benvenuti, F., Stanhope, S. J., Thomas, S. L., Panzer, V. P., & Hallet, M. (1997). Flexibility of anticipatory postural adjustments revealed by self-paced and reaction-time arm movements. Brain Research, 761, 59-70.

Bird, E. I. (1987). Psychophysiological processes during rifle shooting. International *Journal of Sport Psychology, 18,* 9-18.

Bond, J.W. (1995). The individual athlete, In J. Bloomfield & P.A. Fricker & K.D. Fitch (Eds.), Science and medicine in sport (2nd ed., pp.163-190). Australia: Blackwell

Bruner, J. (1990). The act of meaning. Boston, MA: Harvard.

Burton, D. (1989). Winning isn't everything: examining the impact of performance goals on collegiate swimmers cognitions and performance. The Sport Psychologist, 3, 105-132

Cohn, P.J., (1990). Pre-performance routines in sport: Theoretical and practical applications. The Sport Psychologist, 4, 301-312

Cox, R.H., Qui, Y., & Liu, Z. (1993). Overview of sport psychology. In R.N. Singer, M. Murphey, & L.K. Tennant (Eds.) Handbook of research on sport psychology (pp.3-31). New York: Macmillan.

Doss, W., (2003). Train to Win

Engelhorn, R. (1988). EMG and motor performance changes with practice of a forearm movement by children. Perceptual and Motor Skills, 67, 523-529.

Fisher, L.A., Butryn, T.M., & Roper, E.A. (2003). Diversifying (and politicizing) sport psychology through cultural studies: A promising perspective. The Sport Psychologist 17(4), 391-405.

Gauthier, A., Schinke, R.J., Michel, G., Pickard, P., & Guay, M. (2005). Sport psychology research in Northern Ontario, Canada: Cultural and geographic challenges. Paper presented at the meeting of the Canadian Society for Sport Psychology and Motor Learning. Saint Catherine's, Ontario, Canada.

Hardy, J., Gammage, K. L., & Hall, C. R. (2001a). A description of athlete self-talk. The Sport Psychologist, 15, 306-318.

Hardy, J., Hall, C. R., & Alexander, M. R. (2001b). Exploring self-talk and affective states in sport. Journal of Sport Sciences, 19, 469-475.

Hardy, L., Jones, G., & Gould, D. (1996). Understanding psychological preparation for sport: Theory and practice of elite performers. Chichester, UK: John Wiley & Sons.

Kontos, A.P. & Breland-Noble, A.M. (2002). Racial / ethnic diversity in applied sport psychology: A multicultural introduction to working with athletes of color. The Sport Psychologist, 16(3), 296-315.

Krane, V., & Baird, S. (2005). Using ethnography in applied sport psychology. Journal of Applied Sport Psychology, 17(2), 87-107.

Martens, M.P., Mobley, M., & Zizzi, S.J. (2000). Multicultural training in applied sport psychology. The Sport Psychologist, 14(2), 81-97.

Martens, R. (1987). Science, knowledge, and sport psychology. The Sport Psychologist,1(1), 29-55.

Norlander, T., Gård, L., Lindholm, L., & Archer, T. (2003). New Age: Exploration of outlook-on-life frameworks from a phenomenological perspective. Mental Health, Religion & Culture, 6, 1-20.

Pates, J., Cummings, A., & Maynard, I. (2002). The effects of hypnosis on flow states and three-point shooting performance in basketball players. The Sport Psychologist, 16, 34-47.

Pates, J., & Maynard, I. (2000). The effects of hypnosis of flow states and golf performance. Perceptual and Motor Skills, 91, 1057-1075.

Pates, J., Oliver, R., & Maynard, I. (2001). The effects of hypnosis on flow states and golf-putting performance. Journal of Applied Sport Psychology, 13, 341-354.

Ryba, T., Kashope Wright, H. (2005). From mental game to cultural praxis: A cultural studies model's implications for the future of sport psychology. Quest 57, 192-212.

Ryba, T.V., Stambulova, N.B., & Wrisberg, C.A. (2005). The Russian origins of sport psychology: A translation of the early work of A. Tc. Puni. Journal of Applied Sport Psychology 17(2), 157-177.

Salmela, J.H., & Moraes, L.C. (2003). Development of expertise: The role of coaching, families, and cultural context. In J.L. Starkes & K.A. Ericsson (Eds.) Expert performance in sport: Advances in research on sport expertise (pp.275-294). Champaign, IL: Human Kinetics.

Schinke, R.J., & da Costa, J. (2000). Qualitative research in sport psychology. Avante, 6(1), 38-45.

Sparkes, A.C. (2002). Telling tales in sport and physical activity: A qualitative journey. Champaign, IL: Human Kinetics.

Vealey, R. S., & Greenleaf, C.A. (2001). Seeing is believing: Understanding and using imagery in sport. In J. M. Williams (Ed.), Applied Sport Psychology: Personal growth to peak performance (pp. 247-283). Mountain View, CA: Mayfield Publishing Company.

Weinberg, R. S., & Williams, J. M. (2001). Integrating and implementing a psychological skills training program. In J.M. Williams (Ed.), Applied sport psychology: Personal growth to peak performance (4th ed., p. 347-377). Mountain View, CA; Mayfield.

Weinberg, R.S., & Gould, D. (2003). Foundations of sport and exercise psychology (3rd edition). Champaign, IL: Human Kinetics.

INDEX